Luan Ferr

A Practical Manual of Arcturian Healing

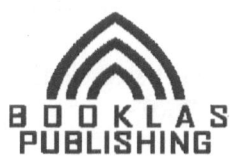

Original Title: Manual Prático de Cura Arcturiana

Copyright © 2025, published by Luiz Antonio dos Santos ME.

This book is a non-fiction work that explores practices and concepts in the field of spiritual healing and multidimensional consciousness. Through a comprehensive approach, the author offers practical tools to achieve energetic balance, holistic well-being, and spiritual expansion.

1st Edition
Production Team
Author: Luan Ferr
Editor: Luiz Santos
Cover Design: Studios Booklas
Typesetting: Emily Harper
Translation: Michael Thompson

Publication and Identification
A Practical Manual of Arcturian Healing
Booklas, 2025
Categories: Spirituality / Holistic Healing
DDC: 133.9013 - **CDU:** 299.93
All rights reserved to:
Luiz Antonio dos Santos ME / Booklas

No part of this book may be reproduced, stored in a retrieval system, or transmitted by any means—electronic, mechanical, photocopying, recording, or otherwise—without prior written permission from the copyright holder.

Summary

Sistematic Index 6
Prologue 12
Part 1 14
1: The Arcturians 14
2: Human Energy Anatomy 25
3: Multidimensional Healing 31
4: The Multidimensional Healing Process 37
5: Cleansing 42
6: Harmonization 46
7: Integration 52
8: Transformation 57
9: Energy Healing 65
10: Regressive Therapy 70
11: Family Constellations 75
12: Meditation 80
13: Creative Visualization 84
14: Affirmations and Decrees 88
Part 2 93
15: The Arcturian Crystals 93
16: Energy Storage 100
17: Elevating Vibration 104
18: Energetic Purification 108
19: Physical Healing 112

20: Emotional Healing 117
21: Mental Healing 122
22: Spiritual Healing 126
Applications of Arcturian Crystals in Healing 130
23: Meditation 130
24: Healing with Hands 134
25: Crystal Elixir 138
26: Crystal Grid 142
27: Chromotherapy with Crystals 146
28: Crystal Programming 151
29: Energetic Cleansing of Spaces 155
30: Chakra Harmonization 159
Part 3 164
31: Sacred Geometry 164
Principles of Sacred Geometry 169
32: Unity 169
33: Patterns 174
34: Golden Ratio 179
35: Vibration 184
36: Symbols 189
37: Healing Codes of Sacred Geometry 195
38: Flower of Life 200
39: Merkaba 202
40: Metatron's Cube 207
41: Spiral 212
42: Mandala 216
43: Meditation with Symbols 221

44: Visualization of Geometric Shapes 225
45: Mandala Construction 230
46: Use of Crystals 235
47: Healing with Hands 239
48: Frequencies of Light and Sound 244
49: Geometry in Our Life 249
Epilogue 252

Sistematic Index

1 - The Arcturians: Introduces the Arcturians, a highly evolved extraterrestrial civilization from Arcturus, who are dedicated to assisting humanity in their spiritual evolution and healing.

2 - Human Energy Anatomy: Explores the subtle bodies, chakras, meridians, and aura that comprise the human energy system, providing a foundation for understanding multidimensional healing.

3 - Multidimensional Healing: Introduces the principles of multidimensional healing, including interconnection, energy, consciousness, responsibility, transformation, and unconditional love, which guide the Arcturian approach to healing.

4 - The Multidimensional Healing Process: Details the steps involved in the Arcturian multidimensional healing process, including diagnosis, cleansing, harmonization, integration, and transformation.

5 - Cleansing: Explains the process of energy cleansing, which removes negative patterns and blockages from the energy field, promoting balance and well-being.

6 - Harmonization: Discusses the harmonization of the energetic system, ensuring that the chakras and energy flows are balanced and aligned.

7 - Integration: Emphasizes the importance of integrating the harmonized energy into all levels of being, consolidating the effects of multidimensional healing.

8 - Transformation: Explores the transformative aspect of Arcturian healing, where limiting patterns are released, past traumas are healed, and individuals awaken to their true spiritual nature.

9 - Energy Healing: Introduces various energy healing techniques employed by the Arcturians, such as Pranic Healing, Reiki, and Quantum Healing, which balance the chakras and restore vital energy flow.

10 - Regressive Therapy: Explains the use of Regressive Therapy to access past memories, identify the origin of traumas, and promote deep emotional healing.

11 - Family Constellations: Discusses the application of Family Constellations to understand and heal family patterns that influence an individual's life and relationships.

12 - Meditation: Guides the practice of meditation for quieting the mind, balancing emotions, and connecting with inner wisdom, facilitating energy harmonization and spiritual expansion.

13 - Creative Visualization: Explains the use of creative visualization to reprogram the mind, manifest healing, and create realities aligned with well-being.

14 - Affirmations and Decrees: Introduces the practice of affirmations and decrees to reprogram the subconscious mind and replace limiting beliefs with positive thoughts.

15 - The Arcturian Crystals: Explores the use of Arcturian crystals as vibrational amplifiers and conductors, enhancing energy healing and harmonization.

16 - Energy Storage: Explains how to store specific intentions and energies within Arcturian crystals for personal use or to assist others.

17 - Elevating Vibration: Discusses the use of Arcturian crystals to elevate the vibration of individuals and environments, facilitating connection with higher dimensions.

18 - Energetic Purification: Explains how to use Arcturian crystals to cleanse the aura, chakras, and spaces, creating a harmonious energy field.

19 - Physical Healing: Explores the application of Arcturian crystals to treat physical ailments, promoting energetic balance and physical well-being.

20 - Emotional Healing: Discusses the use of Arcturian crystals to release traumas, fears, and emotional blockages, promoting emotional balance and self-love.

21 - Mental Healing: Explains how Arcturian crystals can aid in mental clarity, concentration, creativity, and overcoming negative thought patterns.

22 - Spiritual Healing: Explores the use of Arcturian crystals to facilitate connection with the Higher Self, awaken intuition, and expand consciousness.

23 - Meditation: Guides the use of Arcturian crystals during meditation to amplify energy and deepen the meditative experience.

24 - Healing with Hands: Explains how to use Arcturian crystals in conjunction with hands-on healing to enhance energy flow and promote balance.

25 - Crystal Elixir: Provides instructions on preparing and using crystal elixirs made with Arcturian crystals for physical, emotional, and spiritual healing.

26 - Crystal Grid: Explains how to set up crystal grids using Arcturian crystals to amplify intentions and harmonize environments.

27 - Chromotherapy with Crystals: Explores the combination of Arcturian crystals and colors to harmonize the physical, emotional, and spiritual bodies.

28 - Crystal Programming: Provides instructions on programming Arcturian crystals with specific intentions for healing, protection, or manifestation.

29 - Energetic Cleansing of Spaces: Explains how to use Arcturian crystals to cleanse and purify spaces, removing dense energies and restoring harmony.

30 - Chakra Harmonization: Guides the use of Arcturian crystals to harmonize and balance the chakras, promoting overall well-being.

31 - Sacred Geometry: Introduces the Arcturian understanding of Sacred Geometry as an active tool for interacting with cosmic forces and balancing energy.

32 - Unity: Explores the principle of unity in Sacred Geometry, highlighting the interconnectedness of all existence and its role in energetic harmonization.

33 - Patterns: Discusses the significance of geometric patterns in Sacred Geometry, reflecting the cosmic order and facilitating energetic connection.

34 - Golden Ratio: Explains the Golden Ratio and its manifestation in nature, demonstrating its application in energetic realignment and consciousness elevation.

35 - Vibration: Explores the vibrational essence of Sacred Geometry, demonstrating how geometric forms and sound frequencies can be used for healing and spiritual alignment.

36 - Symbols: Discusses the power of Sacred Geometry symbols, such as the Flower of Life and the Merkaba, as portals of connection to higher dimensions.

37 - Healing Codes of Sacred Geometry: Introduces the concept of Healing Codes within Sacred Geometry, revealing their ability to restore energetic balance and promote healing.

38 - Flower of Life: Delves into the Flower of Life, a sacred pattern that reflects cosmic harmony and facilitates access to profound knowledge about creation.

39 - Merkaba: Explains the Merkaba, a light field that surrounds the body and activates the Light Body, promoting multidimensional healing and spiritual connection.

40 - Metatron's Cube: Explores Metatron's Cube, which contains the five Platonic solids and is used for harmonizing subtle bodies and promoting healing.

41 - Spiral: Discusses the spiral as a symbol of growth and evolution, used to activate DNA, accelerate healing, and connect with universal wisdom.

42 - Mandala: Explains the use of mandalas in meditation and healing practices to harmonize energy, calm the mind, and enhance concentration.

43 - Meditation with Symbols: Guides the practice of meditating with Sacred Geometry symbols to elevate vibration, connect with the Arcturians, and promote multidimensional healing.

44 - Visualization of Geometric Shapes: Explains the practice of visualizing geometric shapes to harmonize subtle bodies, promote healing, and manifest desires.

45 - Mandala Construction: Guides the process of creating mandalas with specific colors and shapes to promote emotional healing and spiritual connection.

46 - Use of Crystals: Explores the combination of crystals with Sacred Geometry to amplify healing energy and direct it toward a specific purpose.

47 - Healing with Hands: Explains the technique of using hands to trace Sacred Geometry symbols over the body to promote energetic harmonization and healing.

48 - Frequencies of Light and Sound: Discusses the use of light and sound frequencies that resonate with Sacred Geometry to enhance healing and harmonize subtle bodies.

49 - Geometry in Our Life: Emphasizes the importance of integrating Sacred Geometry into daily life to align with universal patterns and promote balance.

Prologue

There are books that inform, others that enchant. Some offer momentary relief, while others provoke profound reflections. But few, rare and precious, possess the ability to transform the essence of those who read them. This is one such book.

You didn't find it by chance. Something within you, perhaps a subtle intuition or a silent call, brought you to these pages. And by opening it, you have already begun a journey—not just a reading, but a vibrational experience capable of elevating your consciousness and resonating with the purest essence of your being.

The teachings contained here are not mere words; they are keys that unlock internal doors. Revelations that have long awaited access. You will find yourself enveloped by a knowledge that transcends the rational and penetrates deep layers of your energy, your soul. Ancient healing techniques, cosmic wisdom, and connection with beings of very high vibrational frequency are only the surface of what this book will provide.

What do you feel now? Perhaps a restless curiosity, a sense of familiarity, or an inexplicable calling. This is because truth has its own vibration, and your spirit recognizes it. The Arcturians, beings of light who have accompanied our evolution for millennia, share precise methods here to restore your balance, heal invisible wounds, and awaken your highest potential.

The science of multidimensional healing that you will find in these pages is not a distant theory or an abstract concept. It is a real vibrational technology that interacts directly with your energy and accelerates deep processes of alignment and expansion. In each chapter, you will be guided to explore your energy anatomy, activate your intuition, understand hidden patterns, and unlock layers of consciousness that seemed inaccessible.

Allow yourself. Let go of the resistance of the analytical mind, the limiting beliefs and dogmas that have held your perception until now. This book is an invitation to experience, feel, and live a new energetic reality.

Breathe deeply.

The path has already begun, and you are about to cross a threshold where healing becomes part of your existence, and transformation, a certainty.

Welcome to this journey.

Luiz Santos, Editor

Part 1

1: The Arcturians

The Arcturians are a highly evolved extraterrestrial civilization, originating from Arcturus, the brightest star in the constellation of Boötes, located approximately 36 light-years from Earth. Their history dates back billions of years, long enough for them to develop profound wisdom and a technology unimaginable by terrestrial standards.

Arcturians are often described as slender beings, measuring between 1.20 and 1.50 meters tall, with bluish skin and large almond-shaped eyes that radiate serenity and wisdom. Their hands have only three long, delicate fingers, adapted to interact with energy in a subtle and precise manner.

Unlike humans, they do not depend on verbal communication; their language is essentially telepathic, allowing them to share thoughts, emotions, and knowledge instantly and without barriers. Their messages are clear, full of love and discernment, and often accompanied by subtle energetic sensations that envelop those who receive them in a state of peace and deep understanding.

More than their unique appearance, what truly defines the Arcturians is the high vibrational frequency they carry. They have transcended negative emotions and live in a state of unity and harmony, free from judgments and conflicts. For them, everything in the universe is interconnected, and spiritual evolution is a natural and continuous process that leads to ascension. Their commitment to this journey has made them highly compassionate beings, dedicated to loving service and guidance of those who are still taking the first steps on the path of awakening.

The Arcturian presence on Earth is not recent. For millennia, they have accompanied the evolution of humanity, intervening in a subtle way to assist in the spiritual development of our species. As planetary guardians, their mission is to protect Earth from negative influences and guide those who seek to expand their consciousness. They do not impose their help, as they respect the free will of each being, but they are always available to those who wish to connect and receive their assistance.

The history of the Arcturians goes back to a past so remote that it defies our linear understanding of time. Their civilization flourished on a planet orbiting Arcturus, where, over countless eras, they developed a level of consciousness far beyond material limitations. As they advanced spiritually, they learned to manipulate energy in ways unimaginable by terrestrial standards. Their technologies are not based on dense matter, but rather on vibrational resonance and energetic harmonization. Masters in the art of healing, they dominate the science of frequency transmutation, allowing them to transform unbalanced energies into more subtle and beneficial vibrations.

Throughout their evolutionary journey, the Arcturians understood that true spiritual mastery is not limited to individual development, but expands in the form of service to others. Thus, they became mentors of other civilizations, helping various planets overcome challenges and advance on their ascension path. Their commitment to cosmic well-being has led them to establish a network of interdimensional assistance, where they share their wisdom and their advanced healing techniques with those who are ready to receive them.

The Arcturian mission on Earth is broad and multifaceted. One of their main objectives is to raise human consciousness, awakening us to our true divine nature and the unlimited potential we carry. Through their subtle influence, they inspire the development of values such as love, compassion, and cooperation, encouraging us to abandon patterns based on fear and separation.

Another essential aspect of their mission is healing. The Arcturians use advanced energetic healing technologies, capable of acting on the physical, emotional, and spiritual levels. They operate at frequencies that promote the restoration of balance, assisting in the release of traumas and the harmonization of the body's energy centers. Many people who connect with their energy report experiences of profound renewal, where old blockages are dissolved and a sense of lightness and well-being settles in.

In addition, they play the role of planetary protectors, ensuring that Earth is not influenced by external forces that could compromise its ascension process. They work silently, but effectively, neutralizing dissonant energies and protecting our planet from interference that is not aligned with the greater good.

The Earth's ascension to a new vibrational frequency is an event of great importance in the cosmic context, and the Arcturians are here to assist in this transition. They understand that this change does not occur abruptly, but rather gradually, as the collective consciousness of humanity expands. Therefore, they act by inspiring individuals to seek their own evolution, for they know that the transformation of the planet depends on the transformation of each being that inhabits it.

Although the Arcturians exist in a different dimension from ours, it is possible to connect with their energy and receive their guidance. This connection occurs mainly through meditation, visualization, and the sincere intention to tune in to their high vibrations. During these moments of contact, many people report feeling a subtle warmth, a deep peace, or even perceiving insights and symbolic images that bring answers to internal questions.

The benefits of this connection are vast. In addition to the awakening of intuition and the increase in mental clarity, many experience an elevation of energetic frequency, which facilitates healing processes and accelerates the manifestation of positive changes in life. Others report a gradual awakening of dormant psychic abilities, such as extrasensory perception and the ability to feel subtle energies around them. Above all, connecting with the Arcturians provides a deep alignment with the Higher Self, promoting a sense of serenity and purpose.

However, this connection requires surrender and trust. The Arcturians do not impose their presence, nor their teachings. They respect the rhythm of each individual and patiently wait for each one, by their own choice, to decide to open themselves to this high frequency. This process is delicate and occurs in a subtle way, promoting, over time, an expansion of consciousness and a deeper understanding of the meaning of existence.

Those who report experiences of contact with the Arcturians often describe transformative experiences, where they receive deep healings and insights that alter the way they see life. These experiences are not the privilege of a few, but accessible to anyone who seeks inner growth with sincerity.

To facilitate this connection, it is essential to adopt practices that raise personal vibration, such as meditation, self-knowledge, and attitudes based on compassion. As we tune in to this high frequency, it becomes easier to perceive the subtle signs of their presence and guidance.

The path that unfolds before humanity is an invitation to co-evolution and collaboration. The Arcturians, with their millennial wisdom, extend their etheric hands to remind us of who we really are: beings of light in constant evolution. By accepting this call with an open heart, we can become co-creators of a new reality, where love, compassion, and higher consciousness guide each step. This journey is continuous and deeply transformative, and each conscious choice we make brings us closer to a more harmonious and illuminated future.

Although the Arcturians exist in a dimension beyond our physical perception, interdimensional communication becomes possible when the heart is open, the intention is sincere, and specific practices are adopted with discipline and respect. By connecting with these beings of light, you access an inexhaustible source of wisdom, love, and healing, which can transform your spiritual journey and strengthen your connection with higher planes.

Before starting this connection, it is essential to prepare yourself adequately, adjusting body, mind, and spirit to receive the subtle energies of the Arcturians. The first step is purification. For this, take a relaxing bath, allowing the water to carry away any accumulated tension or negativity. In the environment, use incense or smudge sticks such as white sage, palo santo, or myrrh, spreading their smoke through the rooms while visualizing violet light transmuting dense energies into higher vibrations. If possible, light a blue or violet candle, colors associated with Arcturian energy, and visualize its flame illuminating the space with a protective light.

The next step is to find balance. The practice of meditation is highly recommended as it helps to align the energy centers and calm the mind, making communication more fluid. Conscious breathing exercises are also useful: inhale deeply through your nose, hold the air for a few seconds, and then exhale slowly through your mouth, repeating this process until you feel relaxed and centered. Other practices such as yoga, tai chi, or simply walking in nature can help harmonize the body and spirit, preparing you for a deeper connection.

Setting a clear intention is fundamental. Ask yourself what you seek by connecting with the Arcturians: do you desire healing, spiritual guidance, expansion of consciousness, or simply to feel their presence? Formulate this intention objectively and sincerely, expressing it in words or writing it in a spiritual diary. Clarity of purpose facilitates the reception of Arcturian messages and energies, creating a more defined channel of communication.

Finally, it is essential to cultivate an open and receptive mind. Free yourself from rigid expectations and judgments, allowing the experience to manifest naturally. The Arcturians can communicate in subtle ways, such as through intuitive thoughts, physical sensations, or even through signs and synchronicities. Trust the process and be attentive to the small changes around you.

There are several ways to establish this connection, and experimenting with different methods can help you discover which resonates best with you. Meditation is one of the most powerful tools. To do this, find a quiet place, sit comfortably, and close your eyes.

Breathe deeply a few times, visualizing a bright blue light descending from the sky and enveloping your entire being. Visualize the Arcturians approaching, emanating love, wisdom, and healing. Feel their presence and, if you wish, mentally converse with them, expressing your desires and opening yourself to receive their messages. Sometimes, the answers come as soft words in the mind, symbolic images, or sensations of deep peace.

Another effective way is invocation, a direct call to the Arcturians, inviting them to approach and share their guidance. You can create your own invocation or use known phrases, always speaking from the heart. Something like: "Beloved Arcturians, I lovingly invite you to approach. I am open to receiving your wisdom, healing, and guidance. May your light envelop my being and my consciousness, assisting me on my spiritual path. Gratitude for your loving presence." This practice can be done aloud or mentally, depending on what feels most comfortable.

Creative visualization is also a powerful method. Close your eyes and imagine yourself inside an Arcturian ship, surrounded by luminous and benevolent beings. Visualize yourself receiving healing energies, valuable information, and subtle teachings. Feel the vibration of these beings flowing through you, filling every cell of your body with love and peace. The more vivid your visualization, the more intense the connection will be.

Automatic writing is an interesting technique for channeling Arcturian messages. Take paper and pen, relax, and mentally ask the Arcturians to communicate through your writing. Let your hand flow freely, without censorship or judgment, allowing the words to emerge spontaneously. Many times, inspiring and profound messages emerge from this process, bringing valuable insights to your journey.

Dreams can also be a channel of communication. Before going to sleep, ask the Arcturians to send messages or guidance during sleep. Keep a notebook next to your bed and, upon waking, write down everything you remember. Many times, the answers come in the form of symbols or situations that, when analyzed, reveal deep meanings.

In addition, the Arcturians often communicate through signs and synchronicities. Pay attention to repeated numerical patterns, songs that play at the right time, unexpected encounters, or any event that seems to have a special meaning. These small signs indicate that your connection is strengthening.

Deepening this connection requires practice and continuous dedication. Creating an altar dedicated to the Arcturians can be a way to intensify the bond. Choose a special place in your home and place crystals such as amethyst, blue quartz, or lapis lazuli, as well as candles and images that represent Arcturian energy. Use this space to meditate, make invocations, or simply tune in to their presence.

Establishing a communication routine is also important. Set aside a few minutes daily to talk with the Arcturians mentally, express your gratitude, and ask for guidance. The more frequent this practice, the stronger the connection will become.

Seeking knowledge about the Arcturians can further enrich your experience. Read books, participate in study groups, attend lectures, and delve into the philosophy of these beings. Constant learning strengthens trust in the process and broadens your understanding of their messages and purposes.

Another essential aspect is to trust your intuition. Arcturian messages usually manifest as a soft inner voice, a feeling of peace, or an inexplicable certainty. By learning to listen and interpret these signs, you will develop an increasingly clear and assertive connection.

Practicing gratitude also strengthens this bond. Thank the Arcturians for their presence and assistance, even when the answers are not immediate. Gratitude opens paths to new experiences and spiritual deepening.

The benefits of this connection are vast. From physical and emotional healing to spiritual awakening, the Arcturian presence assists in energetic alignment, release of blockages, and strengthening of intuition. Over time, this relationship becomes more and more perceptible, bringing guidance, comfort, and a deep sense of belonging to the universe.

As you delve deeper into this journey, remember that each experience is unique and unfolds in divine timing. Trust the flow of this connection, be attentive to the signs, and celebrate every small advance. Thus, the path unfolds with lightness, guiding you with love and wisdom to a more fulfilling existence aligned with your true essence.

As you delve deeper into this journey, remember that each experience is unique and unfolds in divine timing. Trust the natural flow of this connection, allow yourself to learn from each sign and message, and celebrate each advance, however small it may seem. Thus, the path unfolds with lightness, guiding you with wisdom and love towards a fuller existence, aligned with the universal energy of healing and expansion.

2: Human Energy Anatomy

Delving deeper into our journey toward understanding Arcturian healing, we will now explore the fascinating human energy anatomy. Understanding how vital energy flows through our subtle bodies is essential to grasp the principles of multidimensional healing and apply Arcturian techniques more effectively.

Human energy anatomy goes far beyond what the eyes can perceive. It is a complex and interconnected system that transcends matter, manifesting in subtle layers of energy that influence not only the physical body but also our emotions, thoughts, and spiritual connections. Just as our biological organism has organs and systems responsible for its vital functions, the energy body is also composed of structures that regulate and direct the flow of vital energy — called prana, chi, or ki, according to the spiritual and philosophical traditions around the world.

The subtle bodies form this energetic structure and interpenetrate at different levels of vibrational frequency. Each of them plays a specific role in maintaining the balance of the being. The first and closest to the physical is the etheric body, an energy matrix that acts as a mold for the material body. It is responsible for absorbing energy from the environment and distributing it to the organs and tissues, ensuring vitality and support. The emotional body, in turn, is extremely fluid and dynamic, being directly influenced by the person's emotional state. When negative feelings persist, this body may show distortions and blockages, which, over time, can manifest as psychosomatic illnesses.

The mental body is responsible for processing thoughts, beliefs, and reasoning patterns. It is structured according to how each individual perceives and interprets reality. If fed by negative thoughts or limiting beliefs, it can create energy barriers that directly impact emotional and physical health. Finally, the spiritual body represents the connection with higher dimensions of existence, housing intuition, inner wisdom, and contact with the divine. Its strengthening occurs through spiritual development and alignment with the true essence of the being.

Within this energy system, the chakras play a fundamental role. They are centers of reception, transformation, and energy distribution, influencing physical, emotional, and spiritual aspects. There are seven main ones along the spine, each associated with certain functions. The root chakra (Muladhara), located at the base of the spine, governs security, stability, and connection with the earth. A little higher up, we find the sacral chakra (Svadhisthana), related to creativity, sexuality, and emotions. The solar plexus chakra (Manipura), located in the navel region, is linked to personal power, self-esteem, and willpower. In the center of the chest, the heart chakra (Anahata) manifests as the point of balance between the material and the spiritual, representing love, compassion, and empathy.

In the field of communication and expression, we find the laryngeal chakra (Vishuddha), located in the throat. It governs the verbalization of ideas and the authenticity of personal expression. The frontal chakra (Ajna), between the eyebrows, is known as the third eye, the center of intuition and perception beyond the physical senses. At the top of the head, the crown chakra (Sahasrara) connects the individual to the divine, enabling higher states of consciousness and spirituality. The balance of these energy centers is essential, as any blockage can result in physical, emotional, and spiritual problems.

In addition to the chakras, another essential structure of the human energy system is the meridians. These channels function as "highways" through which vital energy circulates, connecting the organs, the chakras, and the entire energy field. In the tradition of Chinese medicine, techniques such as acupuncture are used to stimulate these points and restore energy flow, removing blockages and promoting healing.

The aura, in turn, represents the energy field that surrounds the entire physical body. It expands and contracts according to the vibrations emitted by the individual, reflecting their state of health, emotions, and spiritual level. Reading the aura can reveal imbalances even before they manifest in the physical body, becoming a powerful diagnostic and self-care tool.

Maintaining energy balance is fundamental to ensure a state of integral health. When energy does not flow properly, various symptoms can arise, such as persistent fatigue, chronic diseases, emotional instability, mental difficulties, creative blocks, and relationship problems. Arcturian healing acts directly on these aspects, restoring the harmony of the chakras, cleansing the meridians, strengthening the aura, and stabilizing the subtle bodies.

Various techniques can be applied to restore and maintain this energy harmony. Meditation is one of the most effective, as it calms the mind, balances emotions, and promotes the free flow of vital energy. The practice of yoga is also highly recommended, as, in addition to improving flexibility and physical strength, it works directly with breathing and the circulation of energy through the body. Another powerful technique is Reiki, a form of energy healing that uses the laying on of hands to channel universal energy and promote the balance of the chakras.

Pranic Healing, in turn, uses prana to remove energy blockages and revitalize the auric field. Crystal Therapy uses crystals and natural stones, each with its specific vibrations, to act on the harmonization of the subtle bodies. Aromatherapy is based on the use of essential oils with therapeutic properties, influencing both the physical and energetic fields. Chromotherapy, on the other hand, works with the vibration of colors, using different shades to restore balance. Finally, Somatotherapy uses sounds and vibrational frequencies to reorganize the individual's energy structure, promoting relaxation and healing.

Understanding human energy anatomy allows us to recognize that true healing happens from the inside out, reaching deep levels of the being. When these structures are aligned and harmonized, the physical body responds with vitality, the mind becomes clear, and the emotions stabilize. The application of Arcturian techniques enhances this alignment, allowing a healing process that transcends the physical level and reaches higher dimensions of existence.

By cultivating the balance of the subtle bodies and keeping the chakras and meridians in constant flow, a field conducive to a fuller connection with cosmic energies is created. This alignment not only favors individual well-being but also contributes to the expansion of collective consciousness and the spiritual evolution of humanity. Even small daily practices of energy harmonization strengthen the vibrational field and facilitate the awakening of the true essence.

Thus, taking care of one's energy anatomy is not just an act of self-knowledge but also a gesture of love and responsibility toward oneself and the whole. Integrating the different healing techniques — whether Arcturian or from other traditions — should be a conscious and respectful process with one's rhythm of development. Honoring this path means allowing vital energy to flow freely, sustaining a more balanced, full life aligned with the soul's purpose.

Therefore, taking care of one's energy anatomy is an act of love and responsibility towards oneself and the whole. The integration of healing techniques, whether they are Arcturian or from other traditions, should be done with awareness and respect for one's own rhythm. By honoring this process, each step taken represents a greater approximation to balance and fullness, allowing vital energy to flow freely and sustain a lighter, healthier life aligned with the purposes of the soul.

3: Multidimensional Healing

With the solid foundation built on human energy anatomy and the connection with the Arcturians, we now enter the fascinating universe of multidimensional healing. Prepare to unravel the principles and foundations of Arcturian healing, which transcends the limits of traditional medicine and acts holistically, integrating body, mind, and spirit.

Multidimensional healing is based on the understanding that the human being is a multidimensional being, composed of several subtle bodies that interact and influence each other. Disease, in this context, is seen as an energy imbalance that manifests at different levels of the being, and can express itself as physical, emotional, mental, or spiritual symptoms.

The Arcturians, with their wisdom and advanced technology, master the art of multidimensional healing, acting on the various subtle bodies to restore harmony and the natural flow of vital energy. They use a holistic approach, integrating different techniques and tools to promote the integral well-being of the individual.

Multidimensional healing is based on essential principles that support the Arcturian approach, allowing a deep realignment of the being at its multiple levels. The first of these principles is interconnection, as every aspect of the human being — physical, emotional, mental, and spiritual — is intrinsically linked. When an imbalance occurs at any of these levels, the others are impacted, perpetuating patterns of disharmony. Multidimensional healing, therefore, does not only treat the manifested symptoms but seeks to restore the integral harmony of the being, ensuring that each aspect is in tune with the others.

Energy is the second fundamental principle. For the Arcturians, all illness or discomfort results from an obstruction or distortion in the flow of vital energy. Through specialized techniques, they remove these blockages, promote the harmonization of the chakras, and restore the body's natural energy flow. By dissolving these energy barriers, the person experiences a return to vitality and balance, allowing their energy to flow freely and sustain health fully.

Consciousness plays an essential role in multidimensional healing. It is through it that the person becomes able to identify patterns of thought, emotions, and behaviors that contribute to their state of imbalance. Self-knowledge, then, becomes a powerful tool within this process, for, by understanding the origins of their disharmony, the person assumes the role of co-creator of their healing. The Arcturians encourage this expansion of consciousness, stimulating each being to develop a deeper perception of themselves and their connections with the universe.

Another essential principle is responsibility. Healing is not a passive act but an active process that demands participation and commitment. The person is invited to take full responsibility for their health, understanding that their daily choices — whether physical, emotional, or spiritual — directly impact their state of balance. The Arcturians teach that self-healing is a path of empowerment with which each being becomes aware of their ability to transform their reality and adopt habits that sustain their harmony and well-being.

Furthermore, multidimensional healing is not limited to the elimination of superficial symptoms; it aims at a deep transformation of the being. Through this process, the person can transcend limiting patterns, heal emotional wounds and past traumas, and access their true divine essence. Thus, healing becomes a catalyst for personal and spiritual evolution, promoting an expansion of consciousness that enables a new way of existing in the world.

Finally, the most essential principle of Arcturian healing is unconditional love. This love, emanated by the Arcturians, creates a vibrational field of healing and transformation. It is within this loving energy that the healing processes occur more fluidly and effectively. Unconditional love, combined with compassion and acceptance, creates a safe space for the person to heal at all levels. This field of healing, sustained by love, dissolves blockages, releases stagnant energies, and allows the true essence of the being to flourish.

The Arcturians use various tools to facilitate this multidimensional healing process, combining advanced technology with energetic methods. Among these tools, Arcturian technology, energy crystals, and light and sound frequencies stand out.

Arcturian technology is one of the most sophisticated and effective approaches within multidimensional healing. Designed to act simultaneously on the subtle and physical bodies, this technology dissolves blockages, raises the vibrational frequency, and reestablishes energy harmony. One of the main resources used is the Arcturian Healing Chambers, energetic spaces created for cell regeneration, chakra alignment, and purification of the energy field.

To apply this technology, the first step is preparation and definition of intention. The environment must be calm and free of external interference, allowing energy to flow without obstacles. The person can sit or lie down comfortably, breathing deeply a few times to relax. With a serene mind, they define the intention of the healing, whether for emotional balance, relief from physical pain, or spiritual expansion.

Then, the connection with the Arcturian Healing Chambers begins. The person can visualize themselves immersed in a blue-violet light, feeling a subtle vibration running through their body. They visualize the presence of the Arcturians around them, allowing them to conduct the healing energy. For a few minutes, the energy flows through every cell of their being, promoting deep regeneration.

Another powerful resource is Arcturian crystals, which act as energy amplifiers and facilitate connection with higher frequencies. Crystals such as clear quartz, amethyst, and selenite resonate strongly with Arcturian energy and can be used to remove energy blockages. To use them, the person can hold a crystal in their hands or position it over the chakra corresponding to the area they wish to treat. They then visualize a beam of blue light emanating from the crystal, penetrating their energy field and dissolving negative patterns, thus restoring the natural flow of energy.

Light and sound frequencies are another essential tool within this healing process. Sound and light vibrate at certain frequencies that can reprogram the energy structure and promote deep harmonization. To apply this technique, the person can use binaural sounds, harmonic chants, or mentally intone the sound "OM". This sound vibration resonates throughout the body, helping to dissolve blockages and raise the vibrational frequency. At the same time, one can imagine rays of golden and sky-blue light flowing around the body, adjusting and realigning all the subtle bodies.

Finally, the anchoring and closing stage is essential to consolidate the effects of the healing. The person can visualize themselves enveloped by a sphere of protective white light, ensuring that the absorbed energy is fully integrated. They express gratitude to the Arcturians and themselves for opening up to the healing process. To complete, drinking water and remaining in a state of tranquility allows the assimilation of energies to occur more deeply and stably.

This practice can be applied both individually and for other people, simply by following the same procedure and establishing the intention to channel healing energy to the receiver. Arcturian technology, when used with consciousness and respect, represents a portal for the full restoration of the being, promoting balance, regeneration, and a spiritual expansion that transcends the limits of ordinary perception.

4: The Multidimensional Healing Process

Multidimensional healing is an individual and unique process for each person. However, some steps are common to all healing journeys:

The first step in this Arcturian multidimensional healing process is the diagnosis, which allows for a thorough analysis of the energy field. It allows the identification of blockages in the chakras, harmful emotional patterns, and limiting beliefs that affect the individual's well-being. Through the advanced vibrational technology of the Arcturians and their elevated energetic connection, it becomes possible to perform detailed mapping, providing a targeted and effective approach to restoring balance.

To begin this journey, proper preparation is essential. Before any evaluation, a suitable, quiet, and distraction-free environment should be created. Choosing a place where you can relax without interruptions is fundamental. When sitting or lying down comfortably, the spine should remain straight so that energy flows without restrictions. With eyes closed, take a deep breath three times, inhaling light and exhaling any tension or distraction. At this moment, it is important to define a clear intention for the diagnosis, thinking: I am ready to understand and identify the blockages that need to be healed. This intention serves as a guide for the energetic connection that will be established. If the process is being conducted for another person, guiding them to follow the same steps ensures efficient harmonization and facilitates the perception of energies.

Connection with the Arcturians is an essential aspect of this assessment, as it allows for an expanded perception of the disharmonies existing in the vibrational field. To establish this contact, visualize a sphere of blue-violet light descending gently from above and completely enveloping the body. This light acts as a channel of connection, intensifying the attunement with Arcturian energy. Then, one should think of the presence of one or more of these elevated beings, perceiving their serene and welcoming energy around them. To deepen this attunement, consciousness needs to be expanded, allowing it to connect to a higher informational field. If desired, it can be verbalized, mentally or in a low voice: I ask for the assistance of the Arcturians to identify and understand the energies that need to be healed. If you are guiding another person, you should guide them through this process calmly and clearly, narrating each step so that the experience is fluid and natural.

The next step is the energetic scan, a method that allows you to detect points of imbalance in the physical, emotional, and spiritual body. To do this, imagine a beam of blue light slowly moving through the body, from the top of the head to the feet. During this process, it is necessary to be attentive to the sensations that arise:

heat, tingling, pressure, or any other subtle perception, as these signs indicate areas with energetic blockages. If the analysis is being done on another person, gently pass your hands a few centimeters from their body, feeling variations in temperature or resistance in the energy field. For an even more accurate perception, a transparent quartz crystal can be used, which amplifies sensitivity and facilitates the capture of more subtle vibrational patterns.

With the blockages identified, the stage of decoding the energetic information begins. Each blocked chakra is directly related to specific aspects of life. The crown chakra, located at the top of the head, when blocked, may indicate a weakened spiritual connection. The frontal chakra, also called the third eye, may point to difficulties in mental clarity or a blocked intuition. In the laryngeal chakra, which governs communication, a blockage can manifest as difficulties in expression or repression of the inner voice. The heart chakra, the center of emotions, can reflect unhealed emotional wounds, while the solar plexus chakra, associated with identity and self-esteem, can show insecurity and emotional blockages. The sacral chakra, responsible for creativity and relationships, can demonstrate difficulties in these aspects when misaligned. The root chakra, at the base of the spine, is related to stability and security, being a point of attention for fears and uncertainties.

After identifying the imbalances, it is important to deepen the understanding of these energetic signs. One should reflect on what patterns of thought or negative emotions may be contributing to these blockages. Asking oneself, or asking the receiver: What is this imbalance trying to teach me? can bring valuable insights into the healing process. All perceptions and intuitions obtained should be recorded, as they will serve as a basis for the next steps in the energetic harmonization journey.

Validating the information obtained is an essential step. With the points of imbalance identified, attention should be turned back to these areas and questioned: What do I need to learn from this blockage? If you are assisting another person, it is important to encourage them to share their sensations and perceptions about the patterns identified. In cases of doubt, you can turn to Arcturian assistance again for confirmation, asking mentally: What additional signs can help me better understand this energy? or What can I do to help in this healing process? This continuous contact strengthens clarity and assertiveness in the diagnosis.

To close this stage and prepare for the healing process, visualizing a golden light filling the points of imbalance is a powerful technique. This light brings immediate relief and initiates the process of energetic restoration. Then, gratitude is expressed to the Arcturians for the assistance received, strengthening the spiritual connection. If the process was conducted for another person, the completion can be done with words of encouragement, such as: Now that we have identified the points of imbalance, we are ready to begin the restoration and harmonization of your energy. Finally, drinking a glass of water helps in the integration of information and allows the energy to flow more lightly through the body.

The diagnosis is an essential step, as it provides a deep understanding of the energetic patterns that need to be worked on. With this clarity, the journey of multidimensional healing becomes more effective and transformative, allowing the restoration of energy to occur in a fluid manner aligned with the purpose of balance and well-being.

The diagnosis is an essential step that allows for a deep understanding of the energetic patterns that need to be worked on. With this clarity, the journey of multidimensional healing becomes more effective and transformative.

5: Cleansing

Following the diagnosis of energy blockages, the next essential step in Arcturian multidimensional healing is energy cleansing. This step removes negative patterns, dissolving accumulated densities in the chakras, meridians, and auric field. Cleansing facilitates the restoration of the natural flow of vital energy, promoting balance and well-being on all levels of being.

Before starting the energy cleansing process, it is crucial to prepare the environment and align the intention. Choose a quiet place, free from external interference, allowing the process to occur without distractions. Sit or lie down comfortably, ensuring that your spine remains straight to facilitate the circulation of energy. Close your eyes and inhale deeply three times, absorbing light and exhaling any accumulated tension. As you do this, mentally declare with conviction: "I am ready to release and purify all dense energies and blockages that no longer serve me." If you are assisting another person, instruct them to follow the same steps, reinforcing their intention to heal.

Next, connect with the Arcturians and activate the light of purification. These beings of high vibration work with a blue-violet light capable of dissolving negative patterns and restoring energy harmony.

Imagine this light descending from above, forming a column of purification around you and enveloping your entire body. Feel the presence of the Arcturians, who project this energy upon you, promoting cleansing and re-balancing.

Allow this light to pass through each layer of your auric field, eliminating emotional toxins, dispersing misaligned vibrations, and restoring your energy balance. If you are guiding another person, describe the process clearly and calmly, encouraging them to visualize and feel this purification happening.

With the energy flowing, it is time to perform the energy sweeping technique. This method helps remove accumulations of dense energy in both the physical and subtle bodies. With your hands, make gentle movements around your body, as if sweeping away any stagnant energy residue. Imagine that you are removing a dark mist or worn-out energy threads, dissolving them in the violet light.

Pay attention to the areas where you feel more resistance or a sensation of heaviness, as these points are often the focus of blockages. If you are assisting someone else, pass your hands about 10 cm from the person's body, removing the dense energies and directing them to be transmuted.

The next step involves the purification of the chakras and energy channels, as these centers can accumulate residues that hinder the flow of vital energy. Start with the crown chakra, at the top of your head, visualizing a violet light dissolving blockages in the spiritual connection.

Then, move your attention to the frontal chakra, located between your eyebrows, and imagine a beam of blue light clearing mental confusion and expanding intuition. In the laryngeal chakra, in the throat region, visualize a light blue light flowing, releasing expression difficulties and removing unspoken words. For the cardiac chakra, in the center of the chest, visualize an intense green light, removing grievances and healing emotional wounds.

In the solar plexus chakra, at the height of the abdomen, project golden light to dissipate insecurities and accumulated tensions. Then, in the sacral chakra, located below the navel, feel a vibrant orange light restoring your emotional and creative vitality. Finally, in the root chakra, at the base of the spine, imagine an intense red light purifying fears and strengthening your energy stability.

If you are guiding another person, verbally lead this visualization, helping them to feel each energy center being cleansed and restored.

For an even deeper purification, use the Violet Flame, a powerful tool of energy transmutation. Visualize this violet fire enveloping your entire body, gently burning any disharmonious energy. Feel this flame consuming negative patterns, dissolving heavy emotions, and neutralizing harmful external influences.

If you wish to enhance this process, mentally repeat: "I transmute all misaligned energy into light, harmony, and balance." If you are assisting another person, guide them to visualize this Violet Flame flowing throughout their being, dissolving any remaining blockages.

After cleansing, it is essential to seal and protect your energy field, ensuring that the restored energies remain balanced. Imagine a sphere of golden light forming around you, creating a vibrational shield that prevents the reabsorption of old patterns. Express gratitude to the Arcturians and your Higher Self for the purification process, recognizing the importance of this moment of healing.

If you are guiding another person, ask them to breathe deeply and feel this protection around them, integrating the experience consciously.

To finalize the process, allow yourself a moment of integration. Drink a glass of water to stabilize the newly harmonized energies and rest for a few minutes, allowing your body and mind to assimilate this vibrational renewal. If you are assisting someone else, guide them to remain in silence and introspection for a few moments before resuming their daily activities.

This energy cleansing practice can be performed regularly, promoting the maintenance of the fluidity of vital energy and preventing the accumulation of new blockages. The more frequent the purification, the lighter and more balanced your energy field will remain, providing greater well-being and attunement with higher frequencies.

6: Harmonization

Following the energetic cleansing, the next essential step is the harmonization of the energetic system, ensuring that the chakras and vital energy flows are balanced. This process stabilizes the vibrational field, aligns the subtle bodies, and strengthens the individual to maintain a continuous state of well-being. The Arcturians utilize different frequencies of light, sound, and crystals to restore this harmony.

To begin energetic harmonization, it is crucial to prepare the environment and align your intention with higher frequencies. Choose a quiet and comfortable place where you can relax without interruptions. This could be a reserved space in your home, a special corner with pillows and candles, or even a silent garden. Sit or lie down comfortably, keeping your spine straight so that energy can flow freely. Close your eyes and breathe deeply three times, feeling the air fill your lungs and, as you exhale, releasing any tension or energetic residue that may still be present.

With each breath, imagine yourself being enveloped by a soft golden light, which brings peace and serenity to your energetic field. Meanwhile, mentally affirm with conviction: "I open my energetic field to receive perfect harmonization and restore the balance of my being." If you are assisting another person, instruct them to follow these same steps and ask them to visualize their body being prepared to receive the harmonizing energy, as if a veil of protective and restorative light were completely enveloping them.

The connection with Arcturian energy is one of the fundamental pillars of this process, as it resonates at an elevated vibration of love and balance. To establish this connection, visualize a sphere of blue-violet light gently descending from above, hovering over your head and, little by little, enveloping your entire being. Feel this vibrant energy flowing through every cell of your body, dissolving any trace of blockages or misalignments. With each new wave of this light, perceive your auric field expanding, becoming lighter, brighter, and more radiant.

As this energy stabilizes around you, you can mentally repeat the affirmation: "I am in perfect harmony with my body, mind, and spirit." If you are assisting another person, verbally guide them through this process, describing in detail the descent of the sphere of light and encouraging them to feel the subtle and loving presence of Arcturian energy.

Now, with the harmonizing energy flowing more evenly, it's time to direct it towards the alignment of the chakras, the centers responsible for channeling and distributing vital energy in your body. Start with the crown chakra, located at the top of your head, and visualize a beam of violet light activating and expanding your spiritual connection. Feel this pulsating energy flowing freely, bringing clarity and a deep alignment with your higher essence.

Next, direct your attention to the brow chakra, or third eye, between your eyebrows. Project a light blue light onto this point, allowing it to bring mental clarity, sharpened intuition, and elevated perception. Allow yourself to trust the flow of wisdom that this light awakens within you.

Moving down a little further, visualize the throat chakra, located in the throat, being enveloped by a soft and serene blue light. This energy unlocks your expression and communication, allowing you to express yourself with authenticity and balance.

In the center of your chest, the heart chakra expands into a golden-green glow, radiating love, compassion, and emotional harmony. Feel this energy restoring any emotional wounds and strengthening your ability to give and receive love unconditionally.

Moving to the stomach area, visualize an intense golden light activating the solar plexus chakra. This energy reinvigorates your confidence, dissolves insecurities, and strengthens your connection with your personal power.

Further down, in your lower abdomen, the sacral chakra is enveloped by a vibrant orange light, activating your creativity, pleasure, and emotional balance. Feel this energy awakening your joy of living and bringing fluidity to your emotions.

Finally, the root chakra, at the base of your spine, illuminates with an intense red light, providing grounding, security, and energetic stability. This light strengthens your connection with the Earth and creates a solid foundation for your vital energy.

If you are assisting another person, guide them to visualize each chakra being filled with its respective light, encouraging them to feel the activation and energetic alignment occurring naturally.

To deepen the stabilization of energy, it is possible to resort to the use of high vibrational frequencies, such as sound, light, and crystals. Chanting the sacred sound "OM" or using binaural frequencies helps these energies resonate in every cell of the body, promoting an even deeper harmonization.

In addition, visualize rays of gold and blue light flowing around you, adjusting your vibrational frequency to a state of perfect harmony. If you wish, use specific crystals, such as clear quartz, amethyst, or selenite, placing them on the chakras to amplify and maintain energetic balance.

If you are harmonizing another person, make gentle circular movements with your hands over each chakra, directing subtle energy to promote balance. These movements act as conductors of energy, reinforcing the flow and vibrational stability.

With the chakras aligned and the energy stabilized, it is time to expand the auric field and integrate this new frequency into the physical and subtle body. Visualize your aura expanding gently, transforming into a bright and pulsating sphere around you.

Feel this energy stabilizing, becoming firm and constant, like a mantle of protective light. To consolidate this vibrational state, mentally affirm: "My energetic field is completely aligned and balanced." If you are assisting another person, ask them to imagine their energy expanding in an enveloping and restorative way.

The next step is the sealing of this restored energy, ensuring that the established harmony remains intact. To do this, visualize a sphere of golden light enveloping the entire body, functioning as a protective shield against any negative influences or energetic misalignment.

Express your gratitude to Arcturian energy and your Higher Self for allowing this deep harmonization. If you are guiding another person, encourage them to feel this energetic protection and to keep it active throughout the day, reinforcing this feeling of balance.

Finally, to ensure that this harmonization remains stable and benefits your daily life, drink a glass of water to help integrate the new frequencies into the physical body. Remain in a state of gratitude and silence for a few minutes, fully absorbing the experience.

If you are assisting another person, guide them to maintain this feeling of balance and well-being throughout the day, paying attention to their energy and avoiding influences that may destabilize it.

Practicing this harmonization regularly will allow you to maintain your elevated vibration and aligned with your spiritual essence, creating a continuous state of well-being and connection with the subtle energies of the universe.

Energetic harmonization can be done regularly to ensure a state of continuous well-being. The more frequent the practice, the more the individual will be able to maintain their elevated vibration and aligned with their spiritual essence.

7: Integration

After the harmonization of the energy system, integration is essential to consolidate the effects of multidimensional healing at all levels of being. This process allows the high frequencies absorbed during healing to be incorporated into the physical, emotional, mental, and spiritual bodies, resulting in lasting changes. Integration prevents the individual from returning to old energy patterns and strengthens the connection with higher states of consciousness.

For the harmonized energy to fully integrate, a careful grounding process is essential, allowing the new vibrational frequency to stabilize in the body and consciousness. Choose a quiet place, preferably in contact with nature or where you can touch the ground with your bare feet. Sit or lie down comfortably and breathe deeply three times, allowing each exhale to release tension and each inhale to bring a sense of welcome and presence.

Visualize luminous roots coming out of the soles of your feet, growing gently towards the center of the Earth. Feel this deep connection, as if you were firmly rooting yourself, allowing your physical body to receive and assimilate the new energies safely and in balance. Perceive the stability that this contact provides you, as if you were firmly anchored in your own inner strength. If you are helping another person, guide them to visualize this anchoring and to feel the solidity of this connection, allowing them to strengthen themselves at the physical and energetic level.

As this foundation is established, it becomes important to expand awareness and recognize the changes that are taking place. Close your eyes and allow yourself to feel the subtle vibrations that run through your body, perceiving every nuance of this new frequency. Ask yourself: "What has changed in my energy? What sensations can I identify?" Carefully observe any changes in your emotional, mental, or physical perception. If you are guiding another person, encourage them to share their impressions and reflections on the process, helping them to become aware of the subtle transformations that may be happening.

With awareness awakened to these changes, it is time to harmoniously distribute the new frequency through the different subtle bodies, promoting a balanced vibrational adjustment. Visualize a golden light enveloping your physical body, filling each cell with revitalizing energy. Feel this light regenerating your biological structure, bringing a sense of renewal and balance. Allow this energy to expand to your emotional body, dissolving old patterns and strengthening elevated feelings, such as love, peace, and gratitude.

Let this light flow into your mind, promoting clarity of thought and alignment with your true essence.

Notice how your thoughts become lighter, more coherent with your purpose and your well-being. Finally, feel this energy reach your spiritual body, connecting you more deeply to your Higher Self and to the higher planes. If you are guiding another person in this process, guide them verbally to visualize and feel this energy flow, helping them to harmonize each part of their being.

With this new frequency integrated, it is crucial to program the mind and the energy field to sustain this state of balance. Affirm internally or aloud words that strengthen this connection, such as: "I am completely aligned with my highest energy", "I fully integrate this healing and allow it to transform my life", or "I am a being of light, balance, and expansion". If you are assisting another person, ask them to choose an affirmation that resonates with their process and repeat it a few times, allowing this intention to take root deeply in their consciousness.

To consolidate this transformation, anchoring the healing in the physical body is essential. Drink a glass of water, allowing your body to absorb this new vibration in a fluid and natural way. Move lightly, stretching your muscles and perceiving how your energy adjusts to movement. Choose activities that give you pleasure and well-being, such as walking outdoors, practicing conscious breathing, or simply resting. If you are guiding another person, guide them to avoid intense stimuli immediately after the session and to respect their own rhythm, resting whenever necessary to consolidate the changes.

Finally, to ensure that this new energy remains protected and stabilized, visualize a sphere of golden light around you, sealing and strengthening your newly integrated vibration. Imagine that this sphere forms a protective shield, allowing only elevated and beneficial influences into your energy field. Feel this protection bringing peace and security, ensuring that your energy remains in harmony. Express gratitude to the Arcturians, your Higher Self, and all the forces that facilitated this transformation process. If you are assisting another person, encourage them to visualize this protective sphere and to feel the stability it provides.

Energy integration does not end with the healing session; on the contrary, it must be continuously cultivated in everyday life. Be mindful of the patterns of thought and behavior you want to strengthen, choosing habits that sustain your elevated vibration. Practices such as meditation, balanced eating, and moments of introspection can be great allies in this process. Whenever you feel your energy fluctuating, reconnect with the golden light and reaffirm your commitment to balance and expansion. If you are assisting another person, guide them to incorporate small daily practices that help them keep this connection alive and present.

This integration process is what transforms the healing experience into a concrete reality. The more conscious and present this assimilation is, the deeper the changes will be in daily life, bringing harmony, well-being, and a renewed connection with your highest essence.

Energy integration is the moment when transformation becomes part of the individual's reality. The more conscious and present this assimilation is, the deeper the changes will be in daily life.

8: Transformation

Transformation is one of the most profound stages of Arcturian multidimensional healing. Unlike clearing and harmonization, which restore balance, transformation allows the individual to release limiting patterns, heal past traumas, and awaken to their true spiritual nature. This process not only alters the energy of the being, but redefines the way they interact with the world and manifest their reality.

Transformation begins with a conscious decision to leave behind old patterns and open oneself to a new vibration. This initial commitment is essential, as it is from it that the whole process unfolds.

To begin this journey, choose a quiet place where you can concentrate without interruptions. Sit or lie down comfortably, breathing deeply a few times to relax and calm your mind. Close your eyes and clearly visualize the intention of transformation, stating internally: "I am ready to transform my energy and release everything that no longer resonates with my evolution."

If you are assisting another person, encourage them to formulate their own intention of transformation in a clear and sincere way, as this is the first step to access the energy of change.

As your intention solidifies, it is time to connect with the Arcturian frequencies of expansion. The Arcturians radiate subtle and powerful energies that assist in accelerating this process, promoting energy renewal and raising consciousness. To access this frequency, visualize a column of blue-violet light gently descending from above and enveloping your entire body. Feel this light penetrating each cell, dissolving resistances and activating a new energetic programming aligned with your highest essence.

At this moment, allow yourself to feel the loving presence of the Arcturians around you, offering support and guidance. If you feel like it, verbalize internally: "I gratefully receive the frequencies of transformation and allow my energy to adjust to my highest potential."

If you are guiding another person, lead them to visualize this blue-violet light acting within and around their energy field, allowing them to fully engage in this transforming vibration.

Deep transformation requires that we become aware of the patterns that need to be modified. This moment of self-reflection is crucial for the process to be effective. Ask yourself:

What behaviors, thoughts, or emotions still limit me?

What negative patterns have I been repeating in my life?

What still holds me to the past and prevents me from fully evolving?

If you are assisting someone, encourage the person to share their perceptions and identify the patterns they wish to transform. Sometimes it can be difficult to recognize these blockages, and in this case, mentally ask the Arcturians to bring clarity and insights about what needs to be worked on. Trust that the answers will come, whether through intuitions, sensations, or memories that arise spontaneously.

With the patterns identified, the essential moment of dissolving and releasing them arrives. To do this, visualize an intense and purifying violet flame burning all the limiting beliefs, dense emotions, and energetic blockages you wish to transmute. Imagine these thought-forms disintegrating little by little, transforming into pure light and returning to the universe in its highest form.

If you feel the need, strengthen this release by verbalizing mentally or aloud: "I release everything that no longer resonates with my growth. I open myself to new possibilities and expansion."

If you are guiding another person, help them visualize the energy being transmuted and encourage them to repeat affirmations that strengthen their liberation. This process is powerful and can bring an immediate sense of lightness and mental clarity.

Now that the old patterns have been dissolved, it is necessary to reprogram the energy with new vibrations aligned with your evolution. Visualize a golden light descending upon you, filling every space that was previously occupied by blockages. This light carries with it high frequencies that reconfigure your energy and strengthen new patterns of thought and behavior.

While this golden light permeates your entire being, mentally affirm affirmations that reinforce this new programming, such as:

"I am free to create my reality with love and wisdom."

"My energy is aligned with my evolution and well-being."

"I allow myself to manifest my full spiritual potential."

If you are assisting another person, guide them to repeat internally or externally positive affirmations that resonate with their new vibration. These words, when felt and integrated, help to consolidate the transformation effectively.

To ensure that this transformation is truly anchored in physical reality, breathe deeply and visualize your renewed energy spreading through all the cells of your body. Gently move your hands, feet, and neck, allowing this new vibration to fully integrate into your physical body. This small act of conscious movement reinforces the connection between the energetic and material planes, bringing the transformation to your daily experience.

Express gratitude for the process performed, recognizing the importance of this change in your journey. If you are assisting another person, ask them to also recognize this transformation and express their gratitude. This simple gesture strengthens the high vibration and consolidates the new energetic frequency in everyday life.

Finally, it is essential to sustain and apply this transformation continuously so that its benefits are lasting. Adopt daily practices that reinforce this new vibration, such as meditation, positive affirmations, and moments of conscious connection with the Arcturians.

Avoid returning to old patterns of thought or behavior. If you notice that you are falling back into old energies, resume the process of dissolution and reprogramming to realign your vibration. If you are assisting someone, encourage that person to maintain daily practices that sustain their transformation and to remember the commitment they made to themselves.

Energy transformation is not just an isolated event, but a continuous process of self-discovery and evolution. The more we open ourselves to this change, the more we align with our spiritual essence and the natural flow of the universe. This journey allows us to transcend limitations, reclaim our true identity, and co-create a higher reality.

May the light and unconditional love of the Arcturians guide each step of this path, strengthening your essence and awakening your unlimited potential. Multidimensional healing is not just an abstract concept, but a real and accessible experience to all who are willing to walk this path of ascension and profound transformation.

Energy transformation is a portal to a new state of being. The more the individual opens themselves to this change, the more they will align with their spiritual essence and their evolutionary journey.

Multidimensional healing is a path of ascension that leads to connection with the Higher Self and the realization of true divine nature. By healing the wounds of the past, freeing oneself from limiting patterns, and raising one's vibration, the individual approaches the light and opens oneself to the experience of unity with the cosmos.

The Arcturians are loving guides on this path of ascension, offering their wisdom, their technology, and their healing energy to help humanity awaken to its true nature and co-create a new world of peace, love, and harmony.

By walking the path of multidimensional healing, each step taken represents an opportunity for self-knowledge and evolution. This process is not limited to the elimination of pains or symptoms, but to the deep understanding that each challenge faced carries a valuable lesson. The Arcturians invite us to see adversities as doors to transformation, encouraging the release of limiting patterns and the reconnection with our divine essence. Thus, healing becomes a continuous journey of growth, where mind, body, and spirit align in perfect harmony.

This deep integration is reflected not only in personal well-being, but also in our relationships and in the way we interact with the world. When we heal our internal wounds and raise our vibration, we positively influence everything around us, creating waves of collective healing and transformation. This is the true purpose of multidimensional healing: to be a catalyst for change, not only for oneself, but for all humanity.

Arcturian wisdom reminds us that we are fundamental pieces in the balance of the cosmos and that, by healing ourselves, we contribute to the vibrational elevation of the planet.

Each transformation, however subtle it may seem, leaves deep marks on the path of spiritual evolution. The journey towards the expansion of consciousness demands surrender and trust, for as old patterns dissolve, new possibilities are revealed. This process does not mean the absence of challenges, but rather the renewed capacity to face them with discernment and lightness, understanding that each experience lived contributes to the strengthening of the soul.

By integrating this new vibration into everyday life, the being begins to radiate their light in a more authentic way, inspiring and elevating those around them. Transformation is not an isolated event, but a continuous flow of learning and realignment, in which each conscious choice strengthens the purpose of ascension. The Arcturians teach that, by cultivating inner peace and connection with the divine, we become agents of change for a more harmonious world, where unity prevails over separation.

Thus, the journey of multidimensional healing is revealed as an invitation to awakening, to the memory of who we really are beyond the limitations of time and space. The more we surrender to this call, the closer we get to the pure essence of universal love. May each step on this path be guided by light, wisdom, and the profound certainty that transformation is the first glimpse of a new state of being, where the infinite potential of the soul can, finally, fully manifest.

9: Energy Healing

The Arcturians are masters of various energy healing techniques, such as Pranic Healing, Reiki, and Quantum Healing, which act directly on balancing the chakras and restoring the flow of vital energy. Through these techniques, it is possible to remove energy blockages, revitalize the auric field, and promote integral regeneration of the being. To apply this healing to yourself or others, follow the steps below:

Before starting the energy healing process, it is essential to create a suitable environment and establish a deep connection with the Arcturian frequencies. To do this, choose a quiet and distraction-free place where you can remain in a state of complete concentration. Sit or lie down comfortably, ensuring your body is relaxed. Then, begin conscious breathing: inhale deeply three times, drawing into yourself a golden light that fills your entire being, and exhale slowly and deeply, releasing any accumulated tension. Feel yourself becoming lighter and more centered.

Now, visualize a beam of sky-blue light gently descending from the cosmos. It approaches like an ethereal mantle that envelops your entire body, creating a protective shield around you. This light not only protects you but also raises your vibrational frequency, allowing for a deeper alignment with the healing energies you are about to channel. Feel this connection intensifying, as if your consciousness were expanding beyond physical space, connecting to the pure essence of Arcturian energy.

With this connection established, you can activate your hands to serve as channels of vital energy. Rub them vigorously against each other, generating heat and activating the energy centers located in the palms. This activation enhances your ability to feel and direct the energy. Now, position your hands about 5 to 10 cm above the body – whether your own body or that of another person if you are applying the healing to someone else. Close your eyes and perceive the vibration of the energy flowing through your hands.

Visualize the Arcturian energy manifesting in your hands as a bright and intense blue-golden light. It descends from the cosmos, passes through the top of your head, and travels through your entire being, flowing freely to the palms of your hands. This energetic flow penetrates deeply into the subtle bodies, radiating balance and restoration.

Now that the energy is active, it is time to harmonize the chakras, which are essential energy centers for physical, emotional, and spiritual balance. Start with the crown chakra, located at the top of the head. Visualize a beam of violet light descending and activating this center, strengthening your connection with higher dimensions. Allow this light to expand your spiritual perception and bring clarity to your purpose.

Next, direct your attention to the frontal chakra, located between the eyebrows. Imagine an intense blue light filling this point, stimulating intuition, discernment, and inner vision. Feel your mind opening to new insights and understandings.

In the laryngeal chakra, visualize a light blue light flowing gently, unblocking any resistance to expression and communication. Feel your voice becoming more authentic and aligned with the truth of your heart.

Now, place your hands over the heart chakra, in the center of the chest, and imagine a pink-green light pulsing and expanding. This glow radiates love, compassion, and harmony, dissolving grievances and opening the way for purer and truer connections.

In the solar plexus chakra, channel a vibrant golden light. This energy dissolves emotional blockages, strengthens your confidence, and activates your personal power. Allow this light to expand, creating a sense of security and autonomy.

In the sacral chakra, visualize an intense vibrant orange light flowing and restoring your creativity, pleasure, and vitality. Feel the energy of this center moving freely, bringing balance to your desires and emotions.

Finally, direct your attention to the root chakra, at the base of the spine. Imagine an intense and firm red light, anchoring your energy in the physical plane and strengthening your sense of stability and security. Feel yourself connected to the Earth, rooted and protected.

After harmonizing the chakras, it is essential to remove any residual energy blockages. With your hands in a sweeping position, as if you were gently cleaning the aura, make slow and fluid movements from the top of the head to the feet. Visualize yourself removing any accumulated energetic density and dissolving it in a transmuting violet flame. This flame has the power to transform any negative energy into pure light.

If you are performing the healing on another person, concentrate on removing specific blockages, observing which areas seem denser or more resistant. As you move your hands over these regions, visualize the energy being extracted and directed to a luminous field of pure regeneration.

To conclude the process, it is essential to seal the harmonized energy, ensuring its full integration into the vibrational field. Imagine a luminous shield enveloping the entire body, creating a protective barrier against external influences. This shield of light ensures that the benefits of healing are preserved and continue to act on your energy field over time.

Finally, express gratitude to the Arcturian energy for its loving assistance, as well as to your own body and energy field for receiving this healing. Feel this gratitude expanding and further strengthening your elevated vibrational state.

To complete the integration of the process, drink a glass of pure water and rest for a few minutes. Allow your body and mind to assimilate the renewed energy, feeling yourself light, balanced, and revitalized.

This practice can be performed daily, whether for self-healing or to help others. Always maintain the intention to channel energy with love, purity, and surrender, for it is this sincere connection that enhances the effects of healing. By incorporating this technique into your routine, you create a continuous flow of well-being and inner transformation, allowing your being to resonate at the highest possible vibration.

The practice of energy healing can be performed daily, promoting a continuous flow of well-being and balance. When applying it to others, follow the same steps, always maintaining the intention to channel energy with love and purity. This technique opens paths to inner transformation, allowing the being to resonate at its highest vibration.

10: Regressive Therapy

Regressive Therapy is a technique used by the Arcturians to access past memories, identify the origin of traumas and emotional blockages, and promote deep healing. This approach allows for the release of limiting patterns that influence current life, promoting transformation and expansion of consciousness. To apply this technique to yourself or others, follow the step-by-step instructions below:

Before starting regressive therapy, it is essential to prepare yourself properly for the process, ensuring a safe environment and a clear intention. Choose a quiet place, free from external interruptions, and make sure the lighting and temperature are comfortable. If you are guiding someone else, ask them to sit or lie down comfortably, preferably wearing light and loose clothing to facilitate relaxation.

Next, breathe deeply three times, allowing your body and mind to enter a state of calm and centering. Feel your breath flowing naturally, filling your lungs and bringing serenity. Meanwhile, clearly define the session's intention. Ask yourself: "What do I want to understand or transform?" The intention may be to discover the origin of an emotional blockage, overcome trauma, or understand repetitive patterns in life. If you are guiding someone else, ask them to express their intention aloud or mentally. This definition will help guide the experience productively.

Now, initiate the induction to an expanded state of consciousness, a fundamental step for the subconscious to access hidden memories. Close your eyes and focus on your breathing rhythm, allowing each exhalation to release tensions and worries. Imagine a flow of golden light enveloping your body, warming and relaxing every muscle, from head to toe.

Visualize a staircase of golden light in front of you. Each step represents a deeper level of relaxation and connection with your inner self. Start descending, step by step, feeling lighter and more receptive with each step. If you are guiding someone else, guide them verbally, suggesting that each step takes them to a deeper level of consciousness and safety. Encourage them to trust the experience, allowing the subconscious mind to open effortlessly.

Upon reaching a state of deep relaxation, direct the mind to access significant memories from the past. Ask open-ended questions that allow answers to arise naturally: "What is the first memory that comes to your mind related to this feeling?" or "What image appears when you think of this blockage?" Do not try to force answers; trust the first impression that arises, whether it is a scene, a sensation, or even an abstract symbol.

If you are guiding someone else, encourage them to describe what they see, feel, or perceive, without judgment or resistance. Some memories may emerge in a fragmented way, and this is normal. If the memory seems vague, ask the person to observe more details, focusing on the senses—what they are seeing, hearing, feeling in the body, or emotionally.

After accessing a relevant memory, analyze it to understand its influence on current life. Observe the details of the scene: where you are, who is present, what emotions are awakened. Ask yourself: "How has this experience affected my life?" or "What patterns have arisen from this?" If you are guiding someone else, guide them with similar questions, helping them explore the connection between memory and the challenges they face in the present.

Recognize the emotions involved and allow them to surface without resistance. Fear, sadness, anger, or guilt may emerge, but they do not need to be repressed. Welcome them as part of the healing process. Often, simply bringing the memory to consciousness already initiates a natural process of release and transformation.

Now that the origin of the blockage has been identified, it is time to promote its healing. Visualize the scene being enveloped by a violet light, an energy of transmutation that dissolves all pain and fear, transforming them into learning and love. Feel this light filling every aspect of memory, bringing understanding and liberation.

If necessary, mentally rewrite the memory. Imagine a positive outcome where your past self receives love, protection, and understanding. If the scene involves other people, visualize them also being enveloped by this healing light, allowing any resentment or hurt to be dissolved. If you are guiding someone else, encourage them to forgive themselves and those involved, releasing the stored emotional weight. Forgiveness does not mean justifying what happened but rather freeing oneself from the pain associated with that experience.

After emotional release, it is time to return to the present, bringing the benefits of the experience. Visualize yourself climbing the golden staircase again, step by step, feeling lighter and renewed with each step. If you are guiding someone else, guide them verbally through the return, ensuring they feel safe and balanced.

Upon reaching the top of the staircase, breathe deeply, and as you exhale, open your eyes slowly. Notice the feeling of clarity and tranquility that has settled. Express gratitude for the learning and integrate this healing into your daily life, adopting more positive thoughts and behaviors.

To ensure the transformation is lasting, it is essential to seal the energy field. Visualize a sphere of golden light enveloping your entire being, protecting and strengthening your new vibration. Feel this energy anchoring deeply, stabilizing the internal changes that have occurred.

Drink a glass of water to help stabilize the energy and write down the insights gained during the session. Recording insights will allow for deeper reflection later, as well as assist in tracking progress over time.

Avoid intense stimuli immediately after practice, such as television, social media, or discussions, allowing the subconscious to process the experience peacefully. If possible, remain in silence for a few minutes, feeling the new frequencies that have been activated.

Regressive therapy is a powerful tool for healing traumas and rewriting negative patterns, promoting deep liberation. By practicing it regularly, each session will reveal new aspects of the journey of self-knowledge and expansion, allowing a continuous process of growth and transformation.

Regressive therapy is a powerful tool for healing traumas and rewriting negative patterns, promoting deep liberation. It can be practiced regularly, allowing each session to reveal new aspects of the journey of self-knowledge and expansion.

11: Family Constellations

Family Constellations are a healing technique that helps in understanding the family patterns that influence our lives, allowing the release of energetic entanglements and the healing of relationships. The Arcturians utilize this tool to assist individuals in recognizing hidden dynamics, harmonizing energetic bonds, and restoring balance within the family system. To apply this practice to yourself or others, follow the step-by-step guide below.

Before starting the Family Constellation practice with the Arcturians, it is essential to create a conducive environment and establish a clear intention. Choose a quiet place where you can conduct the session without interruptions. Ensure that the space is clean and energetically balanced; if you wish, you can light incense, use crystals, or play soft music to promote spiritual connection. Next, sit comfortably and close your eyes. Breathe deeply a few times, allowing your mind to calm and your body to relax. This state of relaxation will facilitate the opening of the energetic field and subtle perception.

Now, concentrate on the issue you wish to work on. It could be a specific family conflict, a repetitive pattern manifesting in your life, or an emotional difficulty you feel is linked to your ancestry. Formulate this intention with clarity, as it will serve as a guide for the entire constellation process.

Family Constellations operate through the morphogenetic field, an invisible network that stores the memories and patterns of past generations. To connect with this field, keep your eyes closed and visualize a circle of light around you, symbolizing your energy and that of your ancestors. This light can be the color that resonates most with you, such as gold, blue, or violet. Gradually, imagine the presence of your family members before you. It doesn't matter if you know everyone personally or if some have passed away long ago; their energy is recorded in this field, and your intention is enough to access it. If you are conducting this practice for another person, ask them to do the same, visualizing their family and observing who stands out in this mental image. Allow yourself to feel the energy of this encounter and perceive what emotions emerge at this moment.

With the connection established, turn your attention to identifying the family patterns that influence your life. Observe which family members emerge with greater intensity in your perception. It may be that a specific ancestor presents themselves with greater clarity or that a strong feeling arises when thinking about a certain person or situation. Pay attention to the emotions that accompany these images. Is there sadness, guilt, fear, or resentment? Or perhaps a feeling of exclusion or repetition? Ask yourself internal questions to deepen this investigation: "Is there a pattern of suffering transmitted through generations?", "Is there something unresolved that manifests in my life unconsciously?", "Am I carrying a weight that does not belong to me?" If you are assisting another person, encourage them to freely express the sensations that arise, without fear or judgment. This is a moment of welcoming and recognizing what needs to be healed.

True healing occurs when we are capable of accepting and honoring the past without resistance or guilt. To do this, visualize each ancestor involved in a golden light, representing recognition and gratitude for their history. Regardless of what they have lived or the difficulties they may have faced, they are part of your lineage and contributed to you being here today. If there are feelings of pain or resentment towards someone, breathe deeply and, internally, repeat the words: "I see you, I recognize your history, and I honor your path. Now I choose to follow my own destiny, free from any weight that does not belong to me." These words help to reorganize the energy and bring understanding. If you are guiding another person, encourage them to say similar phrases, allowing healing to occur naturally and spontaneously.

After this recognition, it is essential to release the energetic entanglements that may be causing blockages. Imagine that there are subtle threads connecting you to the members of your family who influence this issue. These threads can represent unconscious loyalties, limiting beliefs, or pains transmitted from generation to generation. Now, visualize a violet light enveloping these threads, dissolving any dense energy and transforming it into learning and love. If you feel a weight on your shoulders or a sensation of imprisonment, breathe deeply and mentally affirm: "I lovingly return what does not belong to me and follow my path in freedom." This practice helps in restoring balance, allowing each one to occupy their proper place in the family structure. If you are guiding another person, guide them in this visualization and encourage them to repeat the affirmations of liberation.

With the energetic bonds reorganized, it is time to harmonize and integrate the changes that have occurred. Visualize a golden light descending from above and filling your entire energetic field, bringing peace, balance, and protection. This light expands, also enveloping your family members, allowing each one to be in their place with respect and love. Feel this harmony settle within you. Express gratitude for this process, for the learning acquired, and for the opportunity of transformation. If you are guiding someone, suggest that they also give thanks and perceive how they feel after the practice.

To finalize the constellation, it is important to close the process consciously and protect your energetic field. Breathe deeply three times, feeling yourself completely present in the here and now. Visualize yourself enveloped by a sphere of protective white light, ensuring that all the reorganized energy remains stable and strengthened. If you have conducted this experience for another person, guide them to do the same and ask them to share their perceptions, as this helps in the assimilation of learning.

This practice can be repeated whenever you feel the need to strengthen energetic bonds and bring more balance to your life. Family Constellations, when applied with consciousness and respect, promote a deep healing, allowing each individual to assume their true place in the family system and live with more lightness and fullness.

Family Constellations promote a deep healing of relationships and inherited patterns, allowing each individual to assume their true place in the family system. This practice can be repeated whenever necessary to strengthen energetic bonds and bring more balance to personal and spiritual life.

12: Meditation

Meditation is a powerful tool to quiet the mind, balance the emotions, and connect with inner wisdom. The Arcturians use this practice to help with energy harmonization, the awakening of consciousness, and spiritual expansion. Through meditation, it's possible to access elevated states of perception and receive profound insights about the soul's journey. To apply it to yourself or guide it for another person, follow the step-by-step guide below.

Before starting meditation, it is essential to create a suitable environment that promotes relaxation and inner connection. Choose a quiet place where there are no interruptions or noises that could distract the mind. If possible, use elements that help create a serene atmosphere, such as candles, incense, or soft background music. Make sure the room temperature is comfortable, allowing your body to remain relaxed throughout the practice.

Body position also plays an important role in the meditative experience. You can choose to sit with your spine straight, in a comfortable posture, ensuring that your breathing flows freely. If you prefer, you can lie down, as long as you maintain an alert state so you don't fall asleep during the practice. Once you find a comfortable position, gently close your eyes and bring your attention to your breath. Inhale deeply, visualizing the entry of a soft, invigorating light, and exhale slowly, releasing any tension or worry accumulated in the body. Repeat this process a few times, allowing each exhalation to dissolve the tensions and deepen your state of relaxation.

Now, direct your attention to the intention of the meditation. Establishing a clear purpose will help enhance the effects of the practice. Ask yourself: what is the objective of this meditation? Do you wish to achieve relaxation, strengthen your spiritual connection, promote healing, or expand your consciousness? If there is any specific question in your mind, formulate it clearly, allowing the meditation to bring you intuitive insights. To strengthen this intention, visualize a beam of golden light descending from above and enveloping your entire body. Feel this light filling every cell, preparing you energetically for the experience that is about to come.

The breath is the anchor that stabilizes the mind and calms the emotions, allowing you to enter a deeper state of meditation. Start by inhaling slowly through your nose, expanding your abdomen as the air enters. Hold this breath for a few moments, feeling the energy spread through your body, and then exhale gently through your mouth, releasing any residual tension. Continue this cycle for a few minutes, paying attention to the natural flow of air. Each inhalation brings an energetic renewal, and each exhalation releases any blockages that may be present. Let your mind naturally adjust to this rhythm, allowing thoughts to dissolve little by little, without rushing.

At this moment, open yourself to the connection with the Arcturian energy. The Arcturians radiate high frequencies of love, healing, and wisdom, helping to expand consciousness. To tune into this energy, visualize a sphere of bright blue-violet light above your head. This sphere represents contact with the higher planes, a communication channel with beings of high vibration. Imagine this light slowly descending, touching the top of your head and gently expanding throughout your body. Feel this energy filling every part of your being, promoting balance, harmony, and well-being. If you are guiding another person in this process, guide them to visualize this light flowing and enveloping their body, bringing a deep sense of comfort and serenity.

As the mind calms and expands, more subtle perceptions begin to emerge. Allow yourself to enter this state of receptivity, where insights arise naturally. If thoughts or images come to mind, observe them without judgment, as if they were clouds passing in the sky. If you have formulated a question at the beginning of the practice, remain open to receiving intuitive answers. They can come as sensations, symbolic images, or simple inner certainties. Don't force anything, just trust the natural flow of the experience. This is a moment of surrender, where consciousness aligns with higher frequencies, allowing for a deeper understanding of the soul's journey.

When you feel that the meditation is coming to an end, it is important to anchor the energy received and integrate it into your conscious state. Gently bring your attention back to your body, feeling your physical presence and contact with the environment around you. Breathe deeply a few times, moving your fingers and toes slightly. To seal this energy, visualize a golden light enveloping your entire body, like a protective mantle that maintains the high vibrations. If you wish, take a moment to record your perceptions and insights in a notebook, ensuring that you can revisit them later and reflect on your experience.

Finally, remember that meditation is not restricted only to specific moments of practice, but can be integrated into your daily life. Setting aside a few minutes of the day for this connection will strengthen the benefits of meditation over time. Even in the midst of daily activities, you can use conscious breathing techniques to maintain emotional balance and mental clarity. Over time, you will notice subtle changes, such as greater serenity, sharpened intuition, and a deeper connection with universal energy. By making meditation a constant habit, you will open paths to an inner journey rich in self-knowledge, healing, and spiritual expansion.

Meditation is a portal to self-awareness and connection with higher dimensions. Practicing it regularly strengthens inner harmony, promotes mental clarity, and deepens the bond with universal energy.

13: Creative Visualization

Creative visualization is a powerful technique used by the Arcturians to reprogram the mind, manifest healing, and create realities aligned with well-being and spiritual expansion. Through the creation of conscious mental images, it is possible to transform negative patterns and strengthen states of balance and harmony. This practice can be applied to both individual healing and helping others. Follow the step-by-step guide below to use it effectively.

Before starting the practice of creative visualization, it is essential to prepare the body and mind for a receptive state. Choose a quiet environment where you can relax without external interruptions. It can be a silent room, a serene garden, or any space where you feel comfortable and protected. Sit or lie down in a relaxed manner, allowing your body to settle without tension. Close your eyes gently to facilitate concentration and begin to breathe deeply. As you inhale, visualize a golden light filling your lungs, bringing energy and serenity. As you exhale, imagine yourself releasing all accumulated tension, allowing any worry or anxiety to dissolve into the air. Repeat this process a few times until you feel your body and mind in a state of deep relaxation.

With your mind at ease, direct your attention to the intention of the visualization. This is an essential step, as the intention is what guides and strengthens the entire process. Clearly define what goal you want to achieve. It can be the healing of a specific part of the body, emotional balance, the release of energy blockages, or even the manifestation of a desired reality. If you are helping another person, ask what transformation they wish to experience and tune into that intention. Imagine this goal already achieved, feeling in your heart the certainty that the change is in process. The clearer and more vivid this conviction, the greater the impact of the visualization.

Now, with the intention well defined, begin the creation of the corresponding mental image. Imagine a beam of golden light descending from the cosmos and enveloping your entire body or the body of the person being treated. This light is pure healing energy, restoring and balancing every cell, every thought, every emotion. If you are seeking the healing of a specific part of the body, visualize this area being bathed in the regenerating light, which dissolves any blockage or discomfort. If the focus is emotional balance, imagine yourself in a state of deep peace and contentment, as if you were surrounded by a protective aura of serenity and harmony. Allow this image to become more and more detailed and vivid in your mind.

Emotional energy plays a crucial role in the effectiveness of visualization. The more intensely you feel the transformation happening, the faster it will manifest. Bring up feelings of gratitude, love, and joy, as these emotions enhance the energy of the process. Imagine the light expanding, flowing in all directions, and dissolving any trace of resistance or limitation. Feel the relief, the renewal, and the harmony filling your being completely. This is the moment to allow the energy to flow freely, consolidating the healing or desired transformation.

To ensure that the visualization becomes part of reality, it is essential to anchor it in the energy field. Visualize the image created being enveloped by a shield of bright light, like a protection that seals the transformation performed. Reinforce this anchoring by using positive affirmations. Mentally repeat phrases like, "I am completely healed and in perfect harmony" or "The transformation I desire is already manifesting in my life." Allow yourself to feel the truth of these words, incorporating them into your being as part of your new reality. The more deeply this conviction is absorbed, the more lasting the effect of the visualization will be.

Upon completing the practice, it is important to return to the conscious state in a smooth and integrated way. Breathe deeply a few times, feeling your body in the present moment. Move your fingers and toes, gradually bringing your attention back to the environment around you. Open your eyes slowly, allowing the feeling of well-being and balance to settle completely. If you wish, write down your perceptions in a diary, recording your experiences and progress over time. This habit can help you track the evolution of the practice and further strengthen your connection with creative visualization.

The repetition of this technique is essential to consolidate the desired effects. Practice daily, spending at least a few minutes to reinforce the mental image and the energy generated. Whenever you feel doubt or insecurity, return to the visualization to realign your vibration and strengthen your intention. Also, share this practice with other people who seek balance and healing, helping them to transform their realities and expand their own energy field.

Creative visualization is a powerful bridge between the energetic field and manifest reality. The more it is practiced, the more easily the body, mind, and soul align with the desired vibration, allowing healing and transformation to occur naturally and harmoniously.

Creative visualization is a bridge between the energetic field and manifest reality. The more it is practiced, the more easily the body, mind, and soul align with the desired vibration, allowing healing and transformation to occur naturally.

14: Affirmations and Decrees

Affirmations and decrees are powerful tools used by the Arcturians to reprogram the subconscious mind, replacing limiting beliefs with positive and empowering thoughts. When repeated with intention and feeling, these words create new neural connections, aligning the being with a higher vibration of healing and transformation. To use this technique effectively, follow the step-by-step guide below.

Before starting the process of affirmations and decrees, it is essential to establish a solid foundation, starting with a clear definition of intention and purpose. Ask yourself sincerely: "What do I want to transform in my life?" or "What mental pattern do I need to change?" This initial reflection will help guide the practice toward a specific and meaningful goal. If you are helping someone else, encourage them to define a focus, such as healing, self-esteem, or abundance, allowing the intention to be shaped personally and authentically. Clarity is essential for affirmations to have a real and profound impact, as energy follows intention.

After establishing the purpose, it's time to choose and create the appropriate affirmations or decrees. The wording of these phrases should be done positively and in the present tense, as if the desired reality were already happening. The subconscious mind does not recognize negations, so instead of saying "I am no longer sick," the better alternative is "I am healthy and full of vitality." When creating affirmations, opt for short, direct phrases loaded with energetic power, such as:

"My energy is balanced and harmonious." "I am in perfect physical, emotional, and spiritual health." "With every breath, my vitality increases."

If you are guiding someone else in this process, personalize the affirmations according to their specific needs and challenges. In this way, the practice becomes even more effective and meaningful.

The repetition of affirmations should be done with emotion and conviction, because the strength of words is directly linked to the feeling that accompanies them. When repeating the phrases, whether aloud or mentally, get involved with the emotion of what you are affirming. Imagine yourself living the reality expressed by these words, as if the desire had already been realized. This visualization potentiates the reprogramming of the subconscious mind and creates new neural connections aligned with the desired transformation.

A powerful technique to reinforce this practice is the use of the mirror. By looking directly into your own eyes and affirming the phrases with conviction, self-confidence and personal power are intensified. This simple but profound exercise helps dissolve internal blockages and strengthen positive beliefs.

For the practice to have a lasting impact, it is essential to integrate it into daily life. Affirmations should be part of the daily routine, being repeated upon waking and before bed, moments when the mind is more receptive to new information. In addition, writing the phrases and placing them in strategic locations, such as the bathroom mirror, the cell phone screen, or a notebook, helps keep the mind connected to these new patterns of thought.

Another effective way to enhance the effects of affirmations is to associate them with energy practices, such as meditation or conscious breathing. During a moment of introspection, breathing deeply and repeating the phrases allows energy to flow more intensely, facilitating the absorption of messages by the subconscious.

Decrees are an even more powerful tool for deep reprogramming. Unlike affirmations, decrees have an intensified force, being used to create rapid changes in the vibrational field. When making a decree, the voice should be firm and full of authority, charged with intention and certainty. The energy of the word expands when command words are used, such as:

"I AM perfect health and harmony in my body." "By the power of divine light, I decree the complete transformation of my being." "May all misaligned energy be transmuted into love and balance, now!"

If you are guiding someone else in this process, encourage them to pronounce the decrees firmly, feeling the vibration of these words resonating internally. The force with which a decree is expressed directly influences its capacity for manifestation and energetic impact.

After each session of affirmations and decrees, it is essential to allow the integration of the new vibrational frequency. The best way to consolidate this energy is through the feeling of gratitude. After repeating the phrases, pause and feel the transformation happening internally. Express gratitude to the universe, the Arcturians, your Higher Self, or the higher force you believe in, recognizing that the change has already begun to manifest. This simple gesture strengthens the connection with the new energetic pattern and amplifies the effects of the practice.

The continuity of this practice is fundamental for the results to be consistent and lasting. Mental reprogramming happens with the daily repetition of affirmations, and the ideal is to maintain them for at least 21 days, the period necessary for new neural patterns to be established. During this time, adjust the phrases as you feel the need, observing how your mind and your energy evolve.

As the days pass, you will begin to notice subtle changes in your thoughts and emotions. Small signs will indicate that your vibration is adjusting to the new reality you want to create. As your mind aligns with higher frequencies, your external reality will begin to reflect these changes, bringing more balance, inner strength, and full well-being.

Affirmations and decrees are powerful tools of manifestation and healing, as they shape the perception of reality and elevate the vibration of the being. The more they are practiced with intention and emotion, the more deeply they will act in the energetic field, promoting balance, inner strength, and full well-being.

Part 2

15: The Arcturian Crystals

Now that we understand the fundamentals of Arcturian multidimensional healing, it's essential to delve deeper into the relationship between this powerful technique and the energy of crystals. The Arcturians use crystals as vibrational amplifiers, instruments that assist in attuning to higher frequencies and energetic realignment. Through their elevated resonance, crystals facilitate connection with subtler dimensions, allowing healing energy to act even more profoundly and effectively. Let's explore how these energetic tools can enhance transformation and harmonization of being, bringing balance and expansion to those who seek healing at interdimensional levels.

Crystals are powerful tools of healing, used by the Arcturians for millennia to amplify energies, harmonize the subtle bodies, and promote integral well-being.

Crystals are solid structures that form naturally in the Earth's crust, the result of geological processes that combine pressure, temperature, and specific chemical elements. Each crystal possesses a unique molecular structure that determines its energetic and vibrational properties.

The Arcturians, with their advanced technology, cultivate crystals in Arcturus, enhancing their healing properties and programming them with specific frequencies for different therapeutic purposes. These crystals, known as Arcturian crystals, possess a high vibration and an energetic purity that make them exceptional tools for multidimensional healing.

Arcturian crystals possess unique properties that make them highly effective energy amplifiers. Their refined vibrational structure allows them to act in an intensified way in the harmonization of the energy field, raising the frequency of the environments and beings with whom they come into contact. When used correctly, these crystals not only intensify the energies of healing, meditation, and protection, but also serve as powerful conductors, directing energy flows precisely to promote balance and restoration.

In addition to being amplifiers, Arcturian crystals are excellent conductors of energy. They facilitate the passage of vital energy through the subtle bodies, promoting energetic unblockings and restoring the harmony of being. This process can be applied both for one's own well-being and to assist others in the search for balance. To obtain the maximum benefit of this powerful tool, it's essential to know and apply Arcturian crystals correctly, ensuring that their energy is used consciously and effectively.

If the objective is to use the crystals for self-therapy, the first step is the choice of the appropriate crystal for the specific need. The Green Arcturian Crystal, for example, is widely used to promote physical healing, while the Blue Arcturian Crystal aids in relaxation and emotional balance. After selecting the crystal, it's important to prepare the environment in a way that creates a harmonious and tranquil space, where it's possible to lie down or sit comfortably without interruptions. This space should be purified and in tune with the intention of the energetic work.

Before beginning the practice, it's recommended to activate the crystal. To do this, hold it between your hands, close your eyes, and breathe deeply a few times. During this process, concentrate on the energy of the crystal and mentally direct your intention, requesting that it conduct the healing energy to where it's needed. Then, position the crystal directly on the area of the body that needs healing or balance. If the blockage is emotional, it's indicated to position it over the heart chakra, located in the center of the chest. For physical pains or specific discomforts, the crystal should be applied directly to the affected region.

Once positioned, it's essential to visualize the energetic flow occurring actively. Imagine a radiant light emanating from the crystal and gently penetrating the body, dissolving blockages and restoring balance. This process can be intensified through conscious breathing, inhaling deeply and allowing the energy to flow more effectively. The crystal should remain in place for a minimum period of 10 to 15 minutes. During this time, it's advisable to keep the attention turned to physical and emotional sensations, allowing the energy to adjust in a natural way.

At the end of the process, it's important to express gratitude for the healing received. Remove the crystal from the body and hold it again between your hands, recognizing its energetic contribution. If desired, the crystal can be washed under running water or exposed to sunlight for a few minutes for revitalization before the next use. This small closing ritual reinforces the connection with the crystal's energy and enhances its effect for future applications.

In addition to self-therapy, Arcturian crystals can also be used to conduct healing energy to other people. In this case, it's fundamental to follow an appropriate protocol to ensure that the energy is transferred safely and effectively. The first step is the choice of the appropriate crystal for the need of the person who will receive the session. After the selection, the crystal must be cleaned and energized, ensuring that it's free of any previous influences.

Before starting the process, it's essential to ask permission from the person who will receive the energy. Their openness and consent are fundamental for the healing to occur in a fluid way and without resistance. Once authorized, the person should be guided to lie down or sit comfortably and breathe deeply to relax. This facilitates receptivity to the healing energy.

The next step is the activation of the crystal. Holding it between your hands, you must mentalize the intention of directing the healing energy to the person.

With the crystal duly activated, it can be positioned over the area of the body that needs balance or moved gently along the chakras and affected regions. During this process, it's important to visualize the energy flowing from the crystal to the person's body, dissolving blockages and restoring balance.

After 10 to 15 minutes, the crystal should be removed and the person can be invited to share their perceptions about the process. To conclude the session, gratitude is expressed for the energy received and, subsequently, the crystal should be purified before being used again. This final step ensures that the crystal is ready for future applications, without energetic residues from the previous session.

The cleaning and energetic maintenance of Arcturian crystals are fundamental to preserve their effectiveness. Over time, crystals can accumulate dense energies, becoming less efficient. For this reason, it's recommended to clean them regularly using methods appropriate to their composition and properties.

One of the simplest forms of purification is cleaning with running water. This method consists of holding the crystal under filtered water or natural spring water while mentalizing the dissolution of any unwanted energy. To enhance the cleansing, you can mentally affirm that the crystal is being restored to its original vibration. However, it's important to check if the chosen crystal can be wet, as some are sensitive to water.

Another effective technique is cleaning with coarse salt or Himalayan pink salt. For this, simply fill a container with salt and bury the crystal in it for a few hours or overnight. At the end of the process, the salt residues must be removed with a dry cloth or soft brush. This method, however, is not indicated for very porous crystals, which can suffer structural damage.

Smudging with herbs is also an excellent option for purification. Using herbs such as white sage, rosemary, or palo santo, smoke is produced that should be passed around the crystal for a few minutes. During this process, the elimination of any dense energy is visualized, restoring the natural vibration of the crystal.

In addition, energizing through solar or lunar light can be extremely beneficial. For crystals that need intense energization, it's recommended to leave them exposed to sunlight for 1 to 2 hours. For a more subtle and spiritual purification, exposure to the full moon light throughout the night is an excellent choice. However, colored crystals should be protected from direct sunlight, as they can lose their original tonality.

Finally, there is the possibility of using other stones for cleaning. Amethyst and selenite are known for their energetic purification capacity and can be used for this purpose. Simply place the crystal on a druse of these stones and let it rest for a few hours or overnight.

Regardless of the chosen method, the purification of the crystals should be carried out regularly to ensure that their energy is always vibrant and ready to assist in the processes of healing and harmonization. In this way, the Arcturian crystals will remain powerful tools for spiritual elevation and energetic balance.

This method can be repeated whenever necessary to promote healthy energy flow in the body and in the subtle fields.

16: Energy Storage

Arcturian crystals have the ability to store energy, acting as true "energy batteries". This allows them to be programmed with specific intentions, such as healing, protection, prosperity, and ascension, emanating this energy into the environment and to the people around them.

To store energy in an Arcturian crystal, whether for personal use or to assist others, it is essential to follow a careful process that involves choosing, purifying, charging, and stabilizing the energy. This method ensures that the crystal becomes a reliable source of specific vibrations, ready to be accessed whenever necessary.

The first step is to choose the appropriate crystal for the desired intention. Arcturian crystals have different energy frequencies, each attuned to distinct purposes. The green Arcturian crystal, for example, is ideal for promoting physical healing and regeneration, being especially useful for times of convalescence or strengthening the body. The pink Arcturian crystal acts on the emotional field, assisting in self-love and healing emotional wounds, being indicated for those seeking sentimental balance and self-worth. If the intention is prosperity and manifestation of abundance, the golden

Arcturian crystal is the right choice, as it enhances the attraction of opportunities and wealth. For those who wish to improve communication and achieve greater energy balance, the blue Arcturian crystal is recommended, as it resonates with clarity of expression and vibrational harmony. Finally, the violet Arcturian crystal is powerful for purification and spiritual connection, being ideal for meditative practices and elevation of consciousness.

Once the appropriate crystal has been chosen, the next step is to purify it. This process is fundamental to eliminate any pre-existing energies that may interfere with the desired programming. There are several ways to purify, and the choice of method depends on preferences and available resources. An effective option is to wash the crystal in running water, visualizing any unwanted energy being carried away by the water. Another alternative is to use the smoke of sacred herbs, such as sage, rosemary, or palo santo, allowing the smoke to completely envelop the crystal while mentally visualizing its energetic cleansing. Lunar light is also a powerful method, especially if the crystal is left under the full moon light during the night, absorbing its purifying energy.

With the crystal properly cleansed, it's time to energize it with the desired intention. To do this, hold it in your hands and breathe deeply a few times, seeking to enter a state of concentration and connection with your own energy. Close your eyes and visualize an intense light flowing from your hands to the crystal, filling it with the vibration corresponding to the intention you want to store. This light can take on different colors, depending on the purpose: green for healing, pink for love, gold for prosperity, blue for balance, and violet for spiritual purification. During this process, the programming of the crystal can be enhanced by mentally repeating an affirmation, such as: "This crystal is charged with healing and restoration energy." This practice reinforces the intention and anchors the vibration within the crystal.

In addition to visualization and affirmation, there are alternative programming methods that can be used to intensify the connection with the crystal. One of these options is to draw energy symbols on its surface with your finger, imprinting specific meaning on them. Another possibility is to whisper words of intention directly to the crystal, allowing it to absorb the sound vibration of the message. Mantras or chants can also be used to amplify the energetic effect, especially if they are sung in resonance with the vibration of the desired purpose.

After energizing, it is essential to allow the crystal to rest to fully absorb the programmed energy. To do this, choose a sacred place, such as an altar or a special space within your home, and place the crystal there. If desired, you can light a candle near it, symbolizing the activation of its energetic potential. The crystal should remain in this place for a few hours or, preferably, overnight, to ensure that the energy stabilizes and harmoniously settles within its crystalline structure.

Once charged, the crystal can be used in different ways to access its stored energy whenever needed. A simple and effective way is to hold it in your hands in moments of need, allowing its vibration to envelop your body and mind. If you wish to direct the energy to a specific point, simply place the crystal on the corresponding chakra, facilitating the energy transfer to that region. Another option is to place the crystal in an environment, where it will radiate its vibrational frequency into the surrounding space, harmonizing and protecting the place. In addition, the crystal can be shared with another person, allowing them to hold it for a few moments to absorb the energy contained within it.

By following this process, Arcturian crystals become powerful energy storage tools, ready to be activated whenever necessary, offering healing, protection, balance, and vibrational elevation according to the programmed intention.

With this technique, Arcturian crystals become powerful tools of energy available on demand.

17: Elevating Vibration

Arcturian crystals vibrate at high frequencies, helping to elevate the vibration of the environment and people. This process facilitates connection with higher dimensions, the awakening of consciousness, and spiritual healing.

To store energy in an Arcturian crystal, whether for personal use or to assist others, it is essential to follow a careful process that involves choosing, purifying, charging, and stabilizing the energy. This method ensures that the crystal becomes a reliable source of specific vibrations, ready to be accessed whenever needed.

The first step is to choose the right crystal for the intended purpose. Arcturian crystals have different energy frequencies, each attuned to distinct purposes. The green Arcturian crystal, for example, is ideal for promoting physical healing and regeneration, being especially useful for times of convalescence or strengthening the body. The pink Arcturian crystal acts on the emotional field, helping with self-love and healing emotional wounds, being indicated for those seeking emotional balance and self-worth. If the intention is prosperity and manifestation of abundance, the golden Arcturian crystal is the right choice, as it enhances the attraction of opportunities and wealth. For those who wish to improve communication and achieve greater energy balance, the blue Arcturian crystal is recommended, as it resonates with clarity of expression and vibrational harmony. Finally, the violet Arcturian crystal is powerful for purification and spiritual connection, making it ideal for meditative practices and elevation of consciousness.

Once the appropriate crystal has been chosen, the next step is to purify it. This process is essential to eliminate any pre-existing energies that may interfere with the desired programming. There are several forms of purification, and the choice of method depends on preferences and available resources. An effective option is to wash the crystal in running water, visualizing any unwanted energy being carried away by the water. Another alternative is to use the smoke of sacred herbs, such as sage, rosemary, or palo santo, allowing the smoke to completely envelop the crystal while visualizing its energetic cleansing. Moonlight is also a powerful method, especially if the crystal is left under the full moon's light overnight, absorbing its purifying energy.

With the crystal properly cleaned, it is time to energize it with the desired intention. To do this, hold it in your hands and breathe deeply a few times, seeking to enter a state of concentration and connection with your own energy. Close your eyes and visualize an intense light flowing from your hands to the crystal, filling it with the vibration corresponding to the intention you want to store. This light can take on different colors, depending on the purpose: green for healing, pink for love, gold for prosperity, blue for balance, and violet for spiritual purification.

During this process, the crystal's programming can be enhanced by mentally repeating an affirmation, such as, "This crystal is charged with healing and restoration energy." This practice reinforces the intention and anchors the vibration within the crystal.

In addition to visualization and affirmation, there are alternative programming methods that can be used to intensify the connection with the crystal. One such option is to draw energy symbols on its surface with your finger, imprinting them with a specific meaning. Another possibility is to whisper words of intention directly to the crystal, allowing it to absorb the sound vibration of the message. Mantras or chants can also be used to amplify the energetic effect, especially if they are sung in resonance with the vibration of the desired purpose.

After energizing, it is essential to allow the crystal to rest to fully absorb the programmed energy. To do this, choose a sacred place, such as an altar or a special space within your home, and place the crystal there. If desired, you can light a candle near it, symbolizing the activation of its energetic potential. The crystal should remain in this location for a few hours or, preferably, overnight, to ensure that the energy stabilizes and settles harmoniously within its crystalline structure.

Once charged, the crystal can be used in different ways to access its stored energy whenever needed. A simple and effective way is to hold it in your hands in times of need, allowing its vibration to envelop the body and mind. If you wish to direct the energy to a specific point, simply place the crystal on the corresponding chakra, facilitating the energy transfer to that region.

Another option is to place the crystal in an environment, where it will radiate its vibrational frequency to the surrounding space, harmonizing and protecting the place. In addition, the crystal can be shared with another person, allowing them to hold it for a few moments to absorb the energy contained within it.

By following this process, Arcturian crystals become powerful tools of energy storage, ready to be activated whenever needed, offering healing, protection, balance, and vibrational elevation according to the programmed intention.

With this technique, Arcturian crystals help to raise the vibration and promote higher states of consciousness.

18: Energetic Purification

Arcturian crystals have the ability to transmute dense and negative energies into subtle and positive ones. They can be used to cleanse the aura, chakras, and environments, creating a harmonious energetic field conducive to healing.

To apply energetic purification to yourself, the first step is to choose the most suitable Arcturian crystal for this purpose. The Violet Arcturian Crystal is especially recommended for transmuting negative energies and deeply cleansing the aura. If the goal is to achieve a state of calm and emotional balance, the Blue Arcturian Crystal is the best choice. Meanwhile, the White or Transparent Arcturian Crystal is ideal for a broader purification, aligning all chakras and restoring energetic harmony.

Before beginning the process, it is essential to properly purify the crystal so that its energies are clean and ready for use. This can be done using traditional cleansing methods, such as rinsing it under running water, placing it in contact with coarse salt for a few hours, passing it through the smoke of herbs like sage or rosemary, or exposing it to moonlight overnight. After purification, hold the crystal between your hands and mentally set the clear intention to use it to renew your energy, affirming internally: *"This crystal is ready to purify my energy."*

With the crystal prepared, find a quiet place where you can relax without interruptions. Sit or lie down comfortably and take a few deep breaths, allowing your body and mind to enter a receptive state. Hold the crystal in one hand and begin to move it gently around your body, as if sweeping through your aura. Start at the head and slowly move down to the feet. If you sense areas of greater tension or energetic blockages, keep the crystal in those regions for a few seconds, allowing it to work more deeply.

As you perform this movement, visualize a bright light emanating from the crystal—either violet or white—dissolving and transmuting all the dense energy around you. To enhance this effect, mentally repeat affirmations such as: *"All negative energy is being dissolved and transmuted into light."* Feel the lightness and renewal settling into your energetic field.

After about 10 to 15 minutes, conclude the process by placing the crystal over your heart chakra, located at the center of your chest. Take a few deep breaths, feeling your energy restored. Thank the crystal for the purification and store it in a safe place. To complement this internal energetic cleansing, drink a glass of water to help eliminate toxins and promote an even deeper state of balance.

When the intention is to apply purification to another person, it is important to prepare the environment to create a harmonious space conducive to the process. Guide the person to sit or lie down comfortably in a quiet location. To enhance the atmosphere of relaxation and facilitate energetic transmutation, incense, soft music, or candles can be used.

Before beginning, hold the chosen crystal and set the intention for it to serve as a channel of purification for the person's energy. With this clear intention, start moving the crystal around their body, beginning at the top of the head and slowly moving down to the feet. If you sense energetic blockages, keep the crystal over the affected area for a longer time, allowing its vibration to work in dissolving these dense energies.

During the process, visualize the bright light emanating from the crystal, cleansing all energetic impurities from the person. Encourage them to breathe deeply and surrender to the moment, allowing the energy to flow freely. After approximately 10 to 15 minutes, ask them to slowly get up and observe how they feel after the purification. Recommend that they drink a glass of water to enhance the cleansing effect, and finally, purify the crystal before using it again.

When the goal is to purify a space, choosing the right crystal and its strategic placement within the environment are fundamental steps. Ideally, place it in a location where it can radiate its energy widely, such as near the main entrance or at the center of the room.

To activate the crystal's purification power, hold it between your hands and mentally set the intention that it is cleansing and harmonizing the energy of the space. If desired, reinforce this intention by verbalizing affirmations such as: *"This space is free from dense energies and filled with light and harmony."*

In addition to the crystal, the energetic cleansing of the space can be enhanced with complementary techniques. One method is smudging, which can be done with herbs like sage and rosemary. Another option is to pass the crystal through all corners of the space while playing a bell, a Tibetan bowl, or another vibrational sound instrument, as these frequencies further help to dissipate stagnant energies.

To keep the environment harmonized, it is recommended to leave the crystal positioned in the space and repeat the cleansing whenever necessary. Additionally, it is important to recharge the crystal periodically by exposing it to sunlight or moonlight to restore its energy and ensure its continuous effectiveness.

With these practices, Arcturian crystals become powerful allies in energetic purification, removing blockages, dissipating negative vibrations, and restoring balance both in the body and in surrounding spaces.

Through this technique, Arcturian crystals act as true purifiers, removing energetic blockages and restoring harmony.

19: Physical Healing

Arcturian crystals can be used to treat various physical issues such as pain, inflammation, hormonal imbalances, and chronic illnesses. They work on the energetic body, promoting harmonization and rebalancing, which then reflects in physical well-being.

For the application of Arcturian crystals to be effective in restoring and balancing physical health, it is essential to follow a careful and conscious process, whether for personal use or to assist someone else. Interacting with these crystals requires intention, preparation, and connection with the subtle energy they emit.

When using them on yourself, the first step is to choose the appropriate crystal for your specific need. If the goal is cellular regeneration and pain relief, the Green Arcturian Crystal is the best choice, as it directly supports tissue renewal and the dissipation of physical discomfort. If the need is to bring balance and relaxation, especially for relieving muscle tension and inflammation, the Blue Arcturian Crystal is recommended. Meanwhile, the Golden Arcturian Crystal strengthens the immune system and revitalizes the entire body, making it excellent for moments of extreme fatigue or low immunity.

Once the crystal is selected, it is essential to purify it before use. Various energy-cleansing methods can be applied based on preference and availability. Running water is a simple and effective option, allowing the flow of water to wash away any accumulated dense energy. Another alternative is using coarse salt, submerging the crystal in a container with dry salt for a few hours to neutralize negative vibrations. Smudging with herbs such as sage or palo santo is also a powerful practice to restore the crystal's energetic purity. Finally, exposing the crystal to moonlight, especially during the full moon, helps recharge it with subtle and renewing energies. After purification, it is important to hold the crystal in your hands and set the intention for it to be filled with healing energy, visualizing a bright light surrounding the stone and enhancing its therapeutic capacity.

With the crystal ready for use, the next step is to identify the area of the body that requires healing. A brief body scan is recommended: close your eyes, take deep breaths, and focus on perceiving which parts of your body show pain, tension, or any discomfort. This moment of awareness is crucial for directing the crystal's energy with greater precision.

Next, position the crystal directly over the affected area. If dealing with localized pain, such as shoulder tension or abdominal discomfort, simply lie down or sit comfortably and place the stone on the specific region. For more generalized issues, such as extreme fatigue or low immunity, it is advisable to position the crystal over the heart chakra (center of the chest) or the solar plexus chakra (above the navel), as these energy centers play a vital role in physical vitality.

With the crystal in place, the healing energy activation begins. Close your eyes and take deep breaths, allowing yourself to fully relax. Imagine a vibrant light emerging from the crystal and gently penetrating your skin, reaching deeper layers of your body and dissolving any pain or imbalance. To enhance the process, you can mentally repeat a positive affirmation, such as:

"My body is strong, healthy, and in perfect balance."

Repeating this intention strengthens the connection with the crystal and directs its energy toward restoring health.

The ideal duration for this process is approximately 15 to 20 minutes. During this time, focus on the sensations that arise, allowing the crystal to naturally harmonize your body. If you feel any discomfort or restlessness, adjust the position of the stone or simply relax your mind further, letting the energy flow without resistance.

At the end of the process, remove the crystal and express gratitude for the healing energy received. Giving thanks strengthens your connection with the universe and enhances future healing practices. To fully complete the treatment, it is recommended to drink a glass of water, which helps assimilate the energies and promotes an internal sense of renewal. The crystal should be stored in a safe place, and if necessary, the process can be repeated daily until symptoms are alleviated.

When applying healing to another person, the procedure follows similar principles, with some adaptations to provide a more complete and comfortable experience. The first step is to prepare the environment. Ensure that the person is lying down comfortably in a quiet space where they can relax without interruptions. Creating a pleasant atmosphere with soft music or therapeutic aromas such as lavender or lemongrass can further support the process, facilitating relaxation and making the experience even more beneficial.

As with personal use, the choice of crystal should be based on the person's needs, and it must be purified before application. Once the crystal is ready, carefully position it over the affected area or along the main chakras, depending on the situation. If the pain is intense, the crystal can be held close to the area while moving it slowly in circular motions to help disperse accumulated energy and promote a more balanced flow.

During the session, the healing energy can be amplified using the laying on of hands technique. To do this, place one hand over the crystal and the other at the base of the person's spine, creating a more stable and profound energy flow. Visualize the energy flowing through the crystal and filling the person's body with a healing light. This moment is essential for allowing the subtle energy of the Arcturian crystals to work in restoring balance.

After 15 to 20 minutes, remove the crystal and check how the person feels. Ask if there has been any change in their perception of pain or discomfort, and recommend that they rest for a few minutes and drink water to help assimilate the energy received.

Finally, it is important to purify the crystal again before storing it, ensuring that it is ready for future use. By following this process with attention and respect, Arcturian crystals become powerful allies in the pursuit of well-being and bodily harmony, assisting in physical recovery and promoting deep energetic balance.

With this technique, Arcturian crystals serve as powerful tools for restoring physical health, promoting well-being and harmony.

20: Emotional Healing

Arcturian crystals assist in emotional healing, helping to release traumas, fears, and emotional blockages. They promote emotional balance, inner peace, and the development of self-love.

To apply emotional healing to yourself, the first step is to choose the most suitable Arcturian crystal for your current need. If the goal is to strengthen self-love and heal emotional traumas, the Pink Arcturian Crystal is the best choice, as its energy works directly on balancing the heart chakra. If the intention is to calm the mind and reduce anxiety, the Blue Arcturian Crystal is an excellent option, as it soothes thoughts and brings emotional tranquility. For situations involving the transmutation of dense energies and the release of negative emotions, the Violet Arcturian Crystal is the most appropriate, helping to transform limiting emotional patterns.

After selecting the crystal, it is essential to purify and energize it before use. Purification can be done in several ways, depending on your preference. One of the most commonly used methods is cleansing with running water, allowing the flow to wash away energetic impurities. Another effective option is smudging with herbs such as sage or rosemary, letting the smoke surround the crystal and remove any accumulated energetic residues. For those who prefer more subtle methods, moonlight exposure can be used to recharge the crystal—simply leave it out overnight, especially during a full moon. Regardless of the method chosen, when holding the crystal in your hands, set the intention for it to be charged with the energy of emotional healing, visualizing a soft light filling it with positive vibrations.

With the crystal properly prepared, it is time to identify which emotion needs to be worked on. Find a quiet environment where you can sit comfortably and take deep breaths. Close your eyes and allow your feelings to arise without resistance, simply observing them. Ask yourself which emotions are present—it may be sadness, fear, resentment, insecurity, or any other sensation affecting your emotional balance. Acknowledging these feelings is crucial for the healing process to be effective.

After identifying the emotion, place the crystal over the corresponding chakra. If dealing with trauma or emotional pain, position the crystal over the heart chakra, located in the center of your chest. For intense anxiety or deep-seated fears, it is best to place it on the throat chakra or the third eye chakra, located between the eyebrows. If the predominant emotion is insecurity or instability, the crystal can be placed over the solar plexus chakra, just above the navel. Stay comfortable and allow the crystal to work on these energies.

Visualization is an important step to enhance the effect of emotional healing. Close your eyes and imagine a soft light—pink, blue, or violet, depending on the crystal chosen—flowing from the crystal into your body. Visualize this light surrounding the areas where emotional blockages are stored, dissolving tensions and restoring inner harmony. If desired, repeat a healing affirmation mentally or aloud, such as:

"I release my emotional pain and allow healing to take place."

This repetition strengthens your intention and helps reprogram your mind for a more positive state.

Remain in a relaxed state for at least 15 to 20 minutes, allowing the crystal to work energetically. Focus on your breathing, feeling the flow of air entering and leaving your body, and observe any changes in your internal sensations. Some people may feel a slight warmth in the area where the crystal is placed, while others may experience relief or even the release of repressed emotions. All of this is part of the healing process.

At the end of the session, gently remove the crystal and express gratitude for the healing received. A moment of reflection can be valuable after this experience. If you feel the need, write in a journal about the emotions that surfaced, any insights gained, and any significant perceptions that emerged. This practice helps with self-awareness and allows you to track your progress over time. After use, store the crystal in a special place and repeat the practice whenever needed.

When applying emotional healing to someone else, the approach should be equally careful and respectful. First, prepare the environment to ensure the person feels comfortable and relaxed. Choose a quiet space, and if desired, use elements that create a welcoming atmosphere, such as candles, incense, or gentle fragrances. This contributes to a deeper and more restorative experience.

As in self-healing, the choice of crystal should be based on the person's emotional needs. After selecting the appropriate crystal, it must be purified before use, ensuring its energy is clean and ready to work in the other person's energetic field. Once everything is prepared, ask the person to lie down and relax, allowing themselves to enter a receptive state.

The next step is to place the crystal on their body, over the chakra corresponding to the emotion that needs healing. If they are dealing with emotional pain, place the crystal on the heart chakra. If there are blockages related to communication or emotional expression, the throat chakra is ideal. For issues involving intuition and mental clarity, the third eye chakra should be the focus of the energy work.

To activate the healing energy, position your hands above the crystal and visualize a gentle light flowing through it, radiating into the person's energetic field. Encourage them to breathe deeply, inhaling calmness and serenity while exhaling any tension or negative emotions. If they feel comfortable, they can also verbalize positive affirmations, reinforcing their healing intention.

After 15 to 20 minutes, gently remove the crystal and ask the person how they feel. Often, the experience brings immediate relief, but in some cases, deep emotions may continue to be processed over time. Recommend that they drink water to help stabilize their energy, and if possible, rest for a while to integrate the experience more fully.

To complete the process, it is essential to cleanse the crystal after use, ensuring it remains energetically pure for future applications. This can be done using any of the purification methods mentioned earlier, such as running water, smudging, or moonlight exposure.

By following this practice, Arcturian crystals become powerful allies in restoring emotional balance, promoting serenity and well-being for both those who perform and those who receive healing.

21: Mental Healing

Arcturian crystals act on the mental body, aiding in clarity of thought, concentration, creativity, and overcoming negative patterns. They help stabilize the mind and promote a state of intellectual balance.

To apply mental healing to yourself, the first step is to choose the appropriate crystal, as each one has specific properties that directly influence the mind. The Blue Arcturian Crystal is ideal for those seeking to calm the mind and improve communication, while the White or Transparent Arcturian Crystal enhances mental clarity and concentration. The Violet Arcturian Crystal is perfect for those who wish to transmute negative thoughts and strengthen intuition. Choosing the right crystal is essential to correctly direct the energy and achieve the best results.

After selecting the crystal, it is crucial to purify and energize it before use. Purification can be done through different methods, such as rinsing it under running water, placing it on coarse salt, exposing it to moonlight, or using smudging with herbs like sage or palo santo. This process removes any residual energy the crystal may have absorbed. Next, when holding it, one should intend for it to be charged with energies of clarity and mental balance. This moment of connection with the crystal strengthens its purpose and prepares it for practice.

The environment also plays an important role. A quiet and peaceful place should be chosen, where one can sit or lie down comfortably. To facilitate the process, taking a few deep breaths helps relax the body and clear the mind, allowing for better reception of the crystal's energy.

With the environment prepared, it is time to position the crystal on the strategic area of the body. If the goal is to improve focus and concentration, the crystal should be placed on the third eye chakra, located between the eyebrows. If the intention is to dispel negative thoughts and reduce anxiety, the best position is on the crown chakra, at the top of the head. To enhance mental stability and promote a state of emotional balance, the best option is to hold the crystal with both hands at the center of the chest.

When starting the practice, it is important to close the eyes and visualize the energy flowing. Imagine a blue or violet light emanating from the crystal and filling your mind, dissolving dense thoughts and bringing a sense of clarity and harmony. If preferred, this process can be reinforced by mentally repeating a positive affirmation, such as: *"My mind is clear, balanced, and focused."* This step is essential to enhance the crystal's effects and align the mind with the desired energetic frequencies.

The practice should last approximately 15 to 20 minutes. During this period, it is important to focus on the sensation of mental lightness and serenity. The more relaxed and receptive you are, the more effective the absorption of the crystal's energy will be.

At the end, the crystal should be removed calmly, and a moment of gratitude for the process is recommended. This small gesture helps conclude the practice harmoniously. If relevant thoughts or insights arise during the experience, writing them down in a journal can be useful for tracking patterns of mental evolution. The crystal should be stored in a safe place, and the process can be repeated whenever there is a need to restore mental clarity.

To apply mental healing to another person, the first step is to prepare the environment so that it is harmonious and welcoming. A quiet and peaceful place is ideal, and soft background music can be used to enhance relaxation. Creating a space conducive to energetic balance helps the person receive the energy in the purest and most intense way possible.

As in the individual process, choosing the right crystal is essential. The most suitable one for the person's needs should be selected, and before use, purification should be performed to ensure the crystal's energy is clean and ready for application.

With the crystal prepared, the person should lie down comfortably. The crystal should be placed on the third eye if the goal is to stimulate concentration and clarity, or on the crown chakra if the intention is to relieve negative thoughts and bring a sense of lightness. The correct positioning of the crystal allows the energy to be directed effectively.

The activation of mental healing energy is done by keeping the hands above the crystal and visualizing a blue or violet light flowing into the person's mind. This process helps channel the crystal's energy to where it is needed. At the same time, it is important to guide the person to breathe deeply and relax, allowing their energy field to open up to receive healing.

After 15 to 20 minutes, the crystal should be carefully removed. To conclude, it is advisable to ask the person how they feel and suggest that they remain silent and reflective for a few minutes. This moment allows the effects of the practice to be assimilated more deeply.

Finally, the used crystal should be cleansed before being reused, ensuring that it is always energized and ready for a new application. With this technique, Arcturian crystals become powerful allies in restoring mental clarity, promoting a continuous state of peace and balance.

22: Spiritual Healing

Arcturian crystals facilitate the connection with the Higher Self, the awakening of intuition, and the expansion of consciousness. They assist in the ascension journey, promoting spiritual development and a connection with the divine.

To apply spiritual healing to yourself, the first step is to choose the appropriate crystal, as each one has specific properties that facilitate different aspects of spiritual connection. If the goal is to access higher dimensions and promote energetic transmutation, the Violet Arcturian Crystal is the best option. For those seeking to elevate consciousness and strengthen intuition, the White or Transparent Arcturian Crystal is the most suitable. The Golden Arcturian Crystal aids in the expansion of spirituality and alignment with the Higher Self, making it ideal for those who wish to deepen their spiritual journey.

Before using the crystal, it is essential that it is properly purified and energized. This can be done through methods such as exposure to moonlight, rinsing under running water, or smudging with sacred herbs. After purification, hold the crystal in your hands and focus on the intention of charging it with pure spiritual energy. Visualize a bright light surrounding the crystal, enhancing its vibration to support your healing and connection.

Preparing the environment and your own body is a fundamental step to ensure a deep experience. Choose a quiet place where you can be comfortable and free from interruptions. Sit or lie down in a relaxed position and take a few deep breaths, allowing the mind and body to enter a state of calm and receptivity. Conscious breathing is a powerful tool for preparing the energy field and facilitating spiritual connection.

With the environment prepared and the mind at ease, it is time to strategically position the crystal on the body. To enhance the connection with higher dimensions and expand consciousness, the crystal should be placed on the crown chakra, located at the top of the head. If the goal is to activate and strengthen intuition, the crystal can be positioned on the third eye chakra, between the eyebrows. If the intention is to strengthen spiritual presence and the connection with one's essence, hold the crystal with both hands over the heart.

Close your eyes and begin to visualize the energy of the crystal radiating an intense light, which may be violet or golden, filling your body and elevating your vibration. Imagine this light dissolving energetic blockages and opening your consciousness to the spiritual plane. If desired, mentally repeat an affirmation to reinforce the intention of the practice, such as: *"I am connected to my Higher Self and divine wisdom."* Remain in this meditative state for approximately 15 to 20 minutes, allowing the crystal's energy to flow freely.

Observe any sensations, thoughts, or subtle messages that may arise, as they may contain valuable insights for your spiritual journey.

At the end, remove the crystal and express gratitude for the experience and the connection established. If you feel inclined, record in a journal any perceptions, messages, or intuitions that emerged during the practice. This will help track your spiritual evolution over time. Store the crystal in a special place and repeat this process whenever needed, as continuous practice strengthens the connection with higher realms.

If the goal is to apply this technique to another person, the process follows a similar structure with some adaptations. First, it is important to prepare the environment by choosing a quiet and harmonious space. To enhance the experience, incense, candles, or meditative music can be used, creating an atmosphere conducive to spiritual elevation.

With the environment ready, select a crystal suitable for the person's needs and purify it before use to ensure it is free from previous energetic influences. Next, ask the person to lie down comfortably and place the crystal on the crown chakra or third eye, facilitating the connection with higher dimensions and promoting intuitive awakening.

To activate the spiritual energy, position your hands above the crystal and visualize a golden or violet light gently flowing into the person's energy field. Guide them to breathe deeply and relax, allowing the crystal's energy to integrate naturally into their system. During this moment, there may be subtle perceptions, such as an increased sense of lightness or spontaneous mental images, which could indicate important spiritual messages.

After approximately 15 to 20 minutes, remove the crystal and ask the person about their sensations and perceptions. If they received any insights, suggest that they write down their experiences for future reflection. Finally, cleanse the crystal to ensure it is ready for new use.

This practice with Arcturian crystals is a powerful tool for strengthening spirituality, expanding consciousness, and deepening the connection with higher planes, bringing clarity and balance to the spiritual journey.

Applications of Arcturian Crystals in Healing

23: Meditation

Arcturian crystals can be used during meditation to amplify energy, facilitate connection with the Arcturians, and deepen the meditative experience. This practice strengthens inner balance, expands consciousness, and harmonizes the subtle bodies.

To apply this practice to yourself, it is essential to follow a careful process that maximizes the benefits of Arcturian crystals during meditation. The first step is to choose the appropriate crystal for the desired intention. Arcturian crystals possess different energetic properties: the Blue Arcturian Crystal helps achieve inner peace and enhances intuitive connection; the Violet Arcturian Crystal promotes consciousness elevation and the transmutation of negative energies; while the White or Transparent Arcturian Crystal amplifies the connection with higher planes and harmonizes the energy field. Choose the one that best resonates with your current needs.

After selecting the crystal, it is crucial to purify and energize it before the practice. This can be done in various ways, such as rinsing it under running water to eliminate accumulated energetic residues, passing it through the smoke of sacred herbs like sage or palo santo, or leaving it under moonlight to absorb its natural energy. When holding the crystal in your hands, direct your intention for it to act as an amplifier of the meditative experience, connecting you more deeply with your spirituality and inner balance.

The next step involves preparing the environment. Choose a quiet space where you can remain undisturbed. Creating a suitable atmosphere helps enhance the effects of meditation. If desired, light a candle to symbolize inner light or use incense to promote a state of relaxation. Get comfortable, either seated or lying down, ensuring your body is relaxed and aligned.

With the environment prepared, hold the crystal in your hands or place it on one of the body's energy points to intensify its effect. If the goal is to strengthen intuition and mental clarity, place it on the third eye, located between the eyebrows. For higher spiritual connections, position it on the crown chakra, at the top of the head. If you prefer to simply feel the crystal's energy in a subtle way, keep it nearby—on your lap or in front of you—allowing its vibration to integrate into your energy field.

Now, begin the meditation. Close your eyes and take deep breaths, feeling the air entering and leaving your lungs in a serene rhythm. Focus on the presence of the crystal and visualize an intense yet gentle light, which may be blue, violet, or white, depending on the energy of the chosen crystal. This light expands, enveloping your body and bringing a sensation of lightness and deep connection. If desired, mentally repeat an affirmation or mantra, such as: *"I am connected to Arcturian energy, receiving light and wisdom."* Let these words resonate within you, strengthening your energy field.

Remain in this meditative state for as long as you feel necessary, ideally between 10 and 20 minutes. Breathe calmly, observing your thoughts without attaching to them. If you notice your mind wandering, gently bring your attention back to your breath and the presence of the crystal. The key is to stay receptive to the energy and any insights that may arise.

At the end of the meditation, start moving gently, wiggling your fingers and bringing awareness back to your physical body. Open your eyes slowly, allowing yourself to feel the renewed energy. Express gratitude for the crystal and the moment of connection you have just experienced. If you received any significant intuition or sensation, writing it down can be useful for later reflection. Finally, store your crystal in a special place and repeat the practice whenever you wish to strengthen your energy and elevate your vibration.

If the intention is to guide a meditation with Arcturian crystals for another person, the process follows a similar structure with some adaptations. First, create a serene and welcoming environment, ensuring the person feels comfortable. Instruct them to sit or lie down in a relaxed position and close their eyes, breathing deeply to calm the mind and body.

Choose an appropriate crystal based on the person's needs and purify it before use. This process ensures that the crystal's energy is clean and ready to work beneficially. Then, place the crystal on one of the person's energy points. The third eye is ideal for expanding perception and intuition, while the crown chakra facilitates connection with higher dimensions. Alternatively, ask the person to hold the crystal with both hands, allowing them to connect directly with its vibration.

During the meditation, guide the person to visualize a soft light radiating from the crystal and enveloping their entire body. If desired, lead the experience with a calm voice, taking them through a meditative journey that fosters peace and introspection. After about 10 to 20 minutes, instruct them to gradually return to wakefulness, moving their fingers and slowly opening their eyes.

Finally, ask about their experience and encourage reflection on any sensations or perceptions that arose. Cleanse the crystal after use to maintain its pure energy, ensuring it is ready for future practices.

Meditation with Arcturian crystals is a powerful tool for inner balance, vibrational elevation, and consciousness expansion. Whether applied individually or to another person, this practice strengthens spiritual connection and provides a deep state of harmony and well-being.

24: Healing with Hands

Arcturian crystals can be used in conjunction with hands-on healing, amplifying the healing energy and directing it to specific areas of the body. This technique enhances the energy flow, dissolves blockages, and promotes the restoration of physical, emotional, and spiritual balance.

To apply healing to yourself, the first step is to choose the appropriate crystal for your specific need. Arcturian crystals have distinct properties: the Green Arcturian Crystal is ideal for cellular regeneration and physical healing, helping to relieve pain and inflammation; the Blue Arcturian Crystal works on the emotional field, providing relaxation and dissipating tension and stress; while the Golden Arcturian Crystal is a powerful amplifier of vital energy, strengthening the entire energy system and promoting greater vitality.

After selecting the most suitable crystal, it is essential to purify and energize it before use. Purification can be done in different ways, depending on the material and sensitivity of the crystal. Common methods include rinsing it under running water, exposing it to sunlight or moonlight, or smudging it with herbs such as sage or rosemary. When holding the crystal, focus your intention on it serving as a channel to amplify the healing energy, preparing it for the healing process.

Preparing the environment is also a fundamental aspect of ensuring the practice's effectiveness. Choosing a quiet and interruption-free space helps with concentration and connection with the crystal's energy. Elements such as candles, incense, or soft music can be added to enhance the harmonization of the space. Once the environment is ready, find a comfortable position, whether sitting or lying down, ensuring a deep state of relaxation for better absorption of the healing energy.

With everything prepared, begin activating the healing energy. Close your eyes and take a few deep breaths to calm the mind and establish a connection with the energy flow. The crystal should be held in the dominant hand—right for right-handed individuals and left for left-handed individuals—while the other hand is placed over the area of the body that needs healing. At this moment, it is essential to focus on the intention of healing, allowing the energy to flow freely.

Energy is directed through the visualization of a luminous beam emanating from the crystal, passing through the free hand, and reaching the affected area. This energy flow may be felt in different ways, such as a gentle warmth, tingling, or a sensation of lightness. To intensify the process, a positive affirmation can be mentally repeated, such as: *"Healing energy flows through me, restoring my body and balance."* These words help reinforce the intention and enhance the healing effect.

The process should be maintained for about 10 to 15 minutes, allowing the energy to stabilize and fulfill its purpose. During this time, it is important to remain attentive to any sensations that arise, without trying to control them—simply allowing the energy flow to act naturally. Some people may feel immediate relief, while others may notice subtle changes over the following days.

Ending the process should be done respectfully and consciously. At the end of the designated time, express gratitude to the crystal and the energy received, acknowledging the balance and renewal provided. The crystal should be stored safely, and the practice can be repeated whenever harmonization and healing are needed.

When healing is applied to another person, the process follows similar steps but with some important adaptations. The environment should be prepared harmoniously, ensuring the person being treated feels comfortable and relaxed. It is recommended that they lie down or sit comfortably, close their eyes, and take deep breaths to enter a receptive state.

The choice of crystal should be based on the person's specific need. Once the appropriate crystal is selected, it must be purified and energized, just as in the self-healing process. With the crystal ready, the practitioner should position themselves beside the person and begin the energy transfer.

Holding the crystal in the dominant hand, the other hand is placed lightly over the area to be treated, without directly touching the person's body. The energy should be directed consciously and fluidly, using visualization to enhance the process. By imagining the energy flowing from the crystal through the free hand, one should see this force being transferred to the person, promoting well-being and balance. To reinforce the healing intention, a mental affirmation can be repeated, such as: *"Healing energy restores the body and soul, bringing balance and harmony."*

As in self-application, the process should be maintained for about 10 to 15 minutes. During this time, the person may experience different sensations, such as a comforting warmth, deep relaxation, or a gentle vibration in the treated area. At the end of the session, the hands should be removed gently, allowing the energy to settle in the person's body. It is important to give them a few moments to open their eyes and return to full awareness.

After the session, it is advisable to ask the person how they feel and suggest they drink a glass of water to aid in integrating the received energy. Finally, the crystal should be purified again to ensure it remains energetically clean for future uses.

With this practice, hands-on healing combined with Arcturian crystals becomes a powerful tool for balance and renewal. Whether applied to oneself or others, this technique allows access to high-frequency healing energies, promoting harmony in the body, mind, and spirit.

25: Crystal Elixir

Crystal elixirs are prepared with water energized by Arcturian crystals, absorbing their healing properties. They can be ingested or used topically to promote physical healing, emotional balance, and spiritual expansion.

To prepare an Arcturian crystal elixir, the first step is to choose the appropriate crystal based on the intended purpose. Each crystal carries a specific energy that directly influences the effects of the elixir. Among the most recommended, the Green Arcturian Crystal is ideal for promoting physical healing and cellular regeneration. The Blue Arcturian Crystal helps with emotional balance and mental clarity, while the Golden Arcturian Crystal strengthens the energy field and provides revitalization. For those seeking spiritual purification and the transmutation of dense energies, the Violet Arcturian Crystal is the best choice. Lastly, the Pink Arcturian Crystal works on emotional harmony and self-love.

It is crucial to exercise caution when selecting crystals, as not all are safe for direct contact with water. If there is any uncertainty about a crystal's composition or potential toxic elements, it is advisable to use the indirect preparation method to ensure the energetic properties are transferred without the risk of contamination.

Before beginning the preparation, the crystal must be purified and energized to remove any residual unwanted energies. There are several ways to perform this cleansing, such as rinsing the stone under running water, exposing it to the smoke of herbs like sage or rosemary, or leaving it under the moonlight to absorb its energy. After purification, it is important to hold the crystal in your hands and focus on the desired intention, stating something like: *"May this crystal energize the water with healing and balance."* This process enhances the energy transfer to the elixir.

There are two main ways to prepare the elixir: the direct method and the indirect method.

The direct method is only recommended for crystals that are considered safe for immersion in water. To apply it, choose a transparent glass container and fill it with filtered or natural spring water. Place the crystal directly inside the container and position it under sunlight for approximately four hours if you seek energization for vitality and strength. If the goal is a deeper spiritual connection, opt to leave it under the moonlight overnight. Once the energization period is complete, remove the crystal and store the water in a clean glass bottle, ready for use.

The indirect method is safer for crystals that may contain toxic or soluble elements. This process begins by filling a glass container with filtered water. Then, place the crystal inside a smaller glass or within a glass pouch, ensuring it does not come into direct contact with the water. The rest of the process follows the same guidelines as the direct method: exposure to sunlight for four hours promotes vitality, while exposure to the moonlight provides a more subtle and spiritualized energy. At the end of the process, the elixir should be stored in the same way.

Once prepared, the elixir can be used in various ways, with ingestion being one of the most common methods. For internal use, it is recommended to drink a glass of the elixir upon waking or before sleeping, allowing the crystal's energies to be assimilated by the body. It can also be consumed throughout the day as needed to maintain energetic balance. However, it is essential to remember that if there is any doubt regarding the crystal's toxicity, ingestion should be avoided, and the elixir should be restricted to external use only.

For topical application, the elixir can be applied directly to the skin to help relieve inflammation and promote energetic harmonization. A cotton pad soaked in the elixir can be used to cleanse specific areas of the body, such as chakras or regions with energetic tension, facilitating the rebalancing of vital energy.

Another powerful use is as an energy spray, ideal for purifying environments and the aura. To do this, simply transfer the elixir to a spray bottle and use it to energize clothes, objects, or spaces. When sprayed around the body, it helps raise energetic vibrations, providing a sense of lightness and well-being.

To ensure the elixir's durability and effectiveness, it should be stored properly. The ideal method is to keep it refrigerated, which helps preserve its properties and prevents contamination. Consumption should occur within three days to maintain its energetic potency. If an extended shelf life is needed, a few drops of grain alcohol or apple cider vinegar—both natural preservatives—can be added.

With this simple practice, Arcturian crystal elixirs become a powerful tool for vibrational healing, promoting balance in the body, mind, and spirit.

26: Crystal Grid

Crystal grids are geometric formations composed of Arcturian crystals that amplify and direct energy toward a specific purpose, such as healing, protection, manifestation, or energetic balance. They create a powerful vibrational field, enhancing intentions and harmonizing the environment.

To set up an Arcturian crystal grid, it is essential to follow a careful and intentional process, ensuring that energy flows harmoniously and powerfully. The first step is to clearly define the grid's intention. Before assembling it, take a moment to reflect on the specific purpose you wish to achieve. The intention may relate to physical or emotional healing, energetic protection, manifestation of desires and prosperity, or spiritual balance and harmonization. When defining your intention, formulate it as a positive and direct affirmation, such as: "This grid strengthens my energy, promotes healing, and brings harmony around me." This statement will help direct the grid's energy more effectively.

With the intention well established, it is time to choose the most suitable crystals to enhance the desired goal. Arcturian crystals possess different energetic properties, and selecting the right ones will make all the difference. For healing, the Green Arcturian Crystal aids in physical recovery, while the Pink Crystal is ideal for emotional healing. If energetic protection is the focus, the Blue Arcturian Crystal will help create a protective barrier, and the Violet Crystal will work on transmuting negative energies. For manifestation of desires and prosperity, the Golden Arcturian Crystal is the best choice. For spiritual balance, the White or Transparent Arcturian Crystal will help elevate the vibration of both the environment and the person working with the grid.

Before positioning them, the crystals need to be purified and energized. Purification can be done in different ways, such as washing them under running water (preferably from a natural source), placing them under the moonlight, or passing each crystal through the smoke of herbs like sage or palo santo. After cleansing, hold each crystal in your hands, close your eyes, and mentally focus on your intention, infusing them with the energy you wish to manifest through the grid.

The next step is to choose a suitable location for setting up the grid. The space should be calm and free from external interference, such as an altar, a table, or a special corner of the environment. Additionally, the base of the grid can be a fabric with sacred geometry patterns, such as the Flower of Life, the Star of David, or mandalas, or an intuitive pattern can be created, respecting the natural arrangement of the crystals and their connection to the intention.

The arrangement of the crystals follows a specific geometric formation, which helps channel and direct the energy. The first to be positioned is the central crystal, which will be the focal point of the grid and amplify the intention. Then, the remaining crystals are distributed around the central crystal, forming patterns such as triangles, hexagons, or circles. Each formation serves a purpose: the triangle is recommended for manifestation and protection, the hexagon for energetic balance and holistic healing, and the circle for harmony and continuous energy flow. Small crystals can be added between the main points to connect the energies and create a more dynamic flow.

After positioning all the crystals, the grid needs to be activated. To do this, a crystal wand or simply the hand can be used. With gentle movements, pass the wand or fingertips over each crystal, tracing imaginary lines that energetically connect them. While performing this process, visualize a beam of light moving through the grid, linking the crystals and expanding their energy into the environment. If desired, you can reinforce your intention by verbalizing it aloud, further solidifying the grid's purpose.

Once activated, the grid's power can be enhanced through daily meditation beside it, continuously strengthening the programmed intention. It is recommended that the grid remain assembled for at least seven days or until it is felt that its energy has fulfilled its intended purpose. To maintain its effectiveness, activation can be repeated periodically, reinforcing the energy flow.

Maintaining the grid is also an important aspect. Periodically, the crystals should be energetically cleansed to ensure they continue vibrating at their optimal frequency. When it is felt that the grid has completed its role, the dismantling process should be done with gratitude. Remove the crystals one by one, thanking them for the energy shared, and store them carefully for future use. In this way, the Arcturian crystal grid becomes a powerful energy amplifier, assisting in the materialization of intentions and the harmonization of the environment.

27: Chromotherapy with Crystals

Chromotherapy with Arcturian crystals combines the energy of crystals and colors to harmonize the physical, emotional, and spiritual body. Each color possesses a specific vibration that influences the chakras and energetic fields, enhancing healing and balance.

To begin applying chromotherapy with Arcturian crystals to yourself, it is essential to clearly define the purpose of the treatment. Before anything else, reflect on which aspect of your life you wish to harmonize. If the intention is physical healing, the technique will help stimulate cellular regeneration and relieve pain. If the goal is emotional balance, this practice will assist in reducing anxiety, stress, or even overcoming traumas. For those seeking spiritual expansion, the use of colors and crystals can elevate vibration and strengthen the connection with higher planes.

With the purpose well established, the next step is to choose the Arcturian crystals according to their colors and properties. Each crystal emits a specific frequency that directly relates to a chakra, promoting balance and energetic unblocking. The Blue Arcturian Crystal, for example, has a calming vibration that strengthens communication and harmonizes the throat chakra, making it ideal for those who need to express their feelings and ideas more effectively. The Green Arcturian Crystal, in turn, acts directly on physical healing, aiding cellular regeneration and balancing the heart chakra, promoting well-being and vitality. The Violet Arcturian Crystal is known for its ability to transmute negative energies, strengthen intuition, and activate the crown chakra, making it an excellent choice for meditation and spiritual connection. The Golden Arcturian Crystal, on the other hand, amplifies vitality and prosperity, acting on the solar plexus and providing invigorating energy. Finally, the Pink Arcturian Crystal works on self-love and emotional healing, balancing the heart chakra and helping to cultivate feelings of compassion and acceptance.

Before beginning the practice, it is essential to purify and energize the crystals. Choose one of the recommended methods, such as cleansing with running water, which helps remove accumulated energetic impurities; smudging with herbs like sage or palo santo, which purifies and elevates the crystal's vibration; or exposure to moonlight, especially during the full moon, to recharge its energy. When holding the crystal, focus on your intention for the chromotherapy treatment, visualizing the corresponding color filling your energetic field and harmonizing your body and mind.

Chromotherapy application can be performed in different ways, and the choice of method will depend on your preference and current needs. The direct method involves applying the crystal to the body. To do this, lie down comfortably in a quiet environment and place the chosen crystal on the chakra corresponding to the color you wish to work with. Close your eyes and take deep breaths, visualizing the light of the color filling every cell of your body, dissolving blockages, and restoring balance. Stay in this position for about 10 to 15 minutes, allowing the crystal's energy to act subtly and deeply.

If you prefer a method that involves the use of colored light, you can employ a flashlight with a filter of the corresponding color to the crystal. Simply direct the light to the area of the body you wish to treat or illuminate the crystal directly, intensifying its energetic action. While doing this, mentally visualize the color flowing gently and enveloping your aura, promoting balance and well-being.

Another effective approach is the chromotherapy bath, which combines the energy of water with the vibrations of the crystals. For this method, fill a container with pure water and place the chosen crystal inside, leaving it there for a few hours so that the water absorbs its properties. Then, use this water to bathe yourself, washing your face, hands, or body, allowing the revitalizing energy of the crystal to permeate your energetic field. This process is especially recommended for moments of renewal and purification.

Regardless of the chosen method, concluding the practice is an essential step. After applying chromotherapy, express gratitude for the energy received and drink a glass of water to aid in energetic integration. If you feel the need, record your perceptions and sensations in a journal, noting any emotional or physical changes observed during or after the practice.

If the intention is to apply chromotherapy with Arcturian crystals to another person, it is important to prepare the environment in advance. Choose a quiet and peaceful space where the person can relax without interruptions. Soft lighting contributes to a more pleasant experience, and the use of colored candles or fabrics in the tone corresponding to the treatment's intention can enhance the practice's effects.

With the environment prepared, select an appropriate crystal for the person's needs and purify it before use to ensure it is free of residual energies. Then, ask the person to lie down and relax, allowing themselves to surrender to the process. Gently place the crystal on the chakra corresponding to the treatment's objective and, to intensify the energetic flow, use a selenite or white quartz wand, moving it gently over the person's body.

The conduction of chromotherapy energy can be done intuitively. Pass your hands softly over the treated area, visualizing the color flowing through the crystal and enveloping the person in a harmonizing vibration. If desired, use a flashlight with a colored filter to reinforce the effect of the color, projecting its light onto the crystal or directly onto the treated area.

After a period of 10 to 15 minutes, remove the crystal and ask the person about their sensations. Often, they may report feeling lighter, experiencing warmth or coolness in the treated area, or even spontaneous emotional releases. Encourage them to rest for a few minutes and drink water to help enhance the practice's effects. Lastly, remember to cleanse the crystal before reusing it, ensuring it is energetically prepared for future applications.

By incorporating this technique into your routine, chromotherapy with Arcturian crystals becomes a powerful tool for balancing the energetic field and restoring harmony between body, mind, and spirit, providing a profound journey of self-discovery and healing.

28: Crystal Programming

Crystal programming is a technique that allows you to direct the energy of an Arcturian crystal toward a specific purpose, such as healing, protection, prosperity, or spiritual ascension. By programming a crystal, you strengthen your intention and enhance its energetic properties.

To program a crystal for personal use, the first step is to carefully choose the crystal that aligns with your desired intention. Each Arcturian crystal possesses a specific vibration that can be directed toward different energetic purposes. If the goal is to promote physical healing and cellular regeneration, the Green Arcturian Crystal is the ideal choice. For emotional balance and improved communication, the Blue Arcturian Crystal is recommended. If the focus is on energetic transmutation and spiritual protection, the Violet Arcturian Crystal is the most suitable. To attract prosperity and facilitate goal achievement, the Golden Arcturian Crystal can be used. Lastly, to strengthen self-love and assist in emotional healing, the Pink Arcturian Crystal is an excellent option.

Once you have chosen the crystal, it must go through a purification process to remove any previously accumulated energies. This step is essential to ensure effective programming. There are various ways to purify a crystal, and the choice of method may depend on personal preference or the type of crystal. A simple option is to rinse it under running water for a few minutes while visualizing the water washing away all residual energies. Another method is smudging, passing the crystal through the smoke of herbs like sage, rosemary, or palo santo. Exposure to sunlight or moonlight is also an excellent alternative, with sunlight being ideal for intense energization and moonlight for a gentler, more spiritual cleansing.

After purification, it is time to define and enhance the programming intention. Find a quiet place where you can focus without interruptions. Hold the crystal in both hands, take a few deep breaths, and clearly visualize your intention. The formulation should always be specific and positive, as this directly influences the energy stored within the crystal. Some example affirmations include: "This crystal is programmed to promote my healing and energetic balance," "This crystal attracts prosperity and opportunities into my life," or "This crystal strengthens my spiritual protection and purifies my energy."

With the intention well-defined, it is necessary to activate the crystal with your own energy. To do this, close your eyes and visualize a white or golden light emanating from your hands and enveloping the crystal. This light symbolizes the energy being transferred into it. As you perform this visualization, repeat your chosen intention mentally or aloud at least three times. This verbal reinforcement helps solidify the programming within the crystal. To further enhance this activation, you can draw sacred symbols on the crystal's surface, such as the Flower of Life or a Reiki symbol, which are known to amplify energetic vibrations.

After programming, hold the crystal for a few moments and attune yourself to its new energy. This moment is important for feeling your connection with the crystal and ensuring it is aligned with your intended purpose. When storing it, choose a special and secure place, such as an altar, a wooden box, or a velvet pouch, protecting it from external influences. Whenever you feel the need to reinforce the programmed intention, simply hold the crystal again, close your eyes, and visualize its energy flowing in sync with your purpose.

If programming the crystal for someone else, some additional precautions should be taken. The first and most important is obtaining the person's permission, as their receptivity to the crystal's energy directly influences the effectiveness of the programming. Explain the benefits of the technique and ask if they have a specific intention they would like to manifest.

With the person's consent, choose the most suitable crystal for their needs and perform the same purification process mentioned earlier, ensuring it is energetically neutral before programming. Then, hold the crystal between your hands and visualize a golden light surrounding it, symbolizing its energetic activation. While doing this, mentally visualize the person receiving the benefits of the crystal's energy, picturing them in a state of balance and harmony. To strengthen the programming, you can say aloud something like:

"This crystal is programmed to strengthen the energy and assist [person's name] in [specific intention]."

Once the programming is complete, give the crystal to the person and explain how they can best use it. Recommend that they hold the crystal regularly to reinforce their energetic connection with it and keep it in a special, protected place.

To ensure the crystal's programming remains active for extended periods, periodic maintenance is important. This can be done by repeating the activation process whenever needed. Additionally, it is advisable to avoid letting others touch the programmed crystal, as this may interfere with its vibration. If you notice the crystal's energy weakening, a new purification and programming session can be conducted—either to reinforce the original intention or to set a new purpose.

By following these practices, Arcturian crystals become powerful tools for manifestation, aiding in healing, protection, and energetic balance in a personalized way. Conscious and intentional programming of these crystals allows their energies to align with individual needs, making them valuable allies on the path of self-discovery and spiritual evolution.

29: Energetic Cleansing of Spaces

Energetic cleansing of spaces with Arcturian crystals helps remove dense and negative energies, restoring harmony and creating a protected environment conducive to healing and well-being. This technique can be applied to homes, workplaces, or any space in need of purification.

To perform an energetic cleansing with Arcturian crystals, it is essential to follow a careful process that involves selecting the appropriate crystals, proper preparation, and choosing the purification method best suited to the space's needs. This ensures that the location is free of heavy energies and its vibration is elevated, promoting harmony and protection.

The first step is selecting the most suitable crystals for this purpose. The Violet Arcturian Crystal is excellent for transmuting negative energies and raising the space's vibration, while the White or Transparent Arcturian Crystal is ideal for purification and energetic balance. If the goal is to create a serene and protective environment, the Blue Arcturian Crystal is the best choice. Meanwhile, the Golden Arcturian Crystal has the ability to amplify positive energy and strengthen the space's vibrational frequency.

Before using the crystals, it is crucial to purify them to remove any residual accumulated energy. This can be done in various ways. One of the most effective methods is smudging with herbs like sage, rosemary, or palo santo, which have natural purifying properties. Another option is rinsing the crystals under running water, if they are water-resistant, allowing stagnant energy to be washed away. Crystals can also be recharged by exposing them to sunlight or moonlight, ensuring their vibrational strength is at its peak for the energetic cleansing process.

Once the crystals are properly prepared, it is time to choose the most appropriate method for cleansing the space.

One of the simplest and most effective ways is to strategically place crystals throughout the space. Positioning a crystal near the entrance helps block unwanted energies before they enter. Placing crystals in the corners of the room aids in dispersing accumulated energies, while a crystal placed at the center of the space acts as a radiating point of energetic balance. This method is ideal for those who wish to maintain continuous purification, requiring only regular cleansing of the crystals to preserve their potency.

Another powerful approach is actively passing the crystal through the space. To do this, hold a crystal programmed for purification in your dominant hand and walk through the area, moving it through the air in circular or gentle motions. During this process, it is recommended to visualize a violet or white light filling the entire space, dissolving any dense energy present.

To enhance the effect, you can repeat a positive affirmation mentally or aloud, such as: "This space is purified and filled with light and harmony." This method is particularly useful for quick and effective cleansings after draining events, such as arguments or visits from people with heavy energy.

For those who prefer a more subtle and continuous method, a crystal elixir is an excellent alternative. It is prepared by placing an Arcturian Crystal in a container with filtered water for a few hours, allowing the crystal's vibration to infuse the liquid. Then, transfer the elixir into a spray bottle and mist it in the corners of the space, at the entrance, and even on furniture. This method is highly recommended for spaces that feel stagnant or heavy, as it gently and evenly spreads the crystals' vibration.

Another highly effective technique for cleansing and continuous protection is creating a crystal grid. For this, Arcturian crystals previously programmed for purification should be placed around the space, forming a circle or a six-pointed star. This geometric configuration enhances the crystals' energy, creating a vibrational field of protection around the location. To activate the grid, simply visualize a shield of light enveloping the entire space, ensuring lasting energetic balance and security.

Regardless of the chosen method, regular maintenance of energetic cleansing is important. Whenever there are visitors, arguments, or significant changes in the environment, it is recommended to repeat the process to restore harmony. Additionally, the crystals should be periodically cleansed to ensure they continue vibrating at their highest potential.

To further enhance the effects of cleansing, it is beneficial to cultivate habits that keep the space's energy elevated daily. Using incense, keeping plants in the area, and practicing positive intentions while occupying the space are effective ways to maintain a harmonious and protected environment.

By following these steps, Arcturian crystals serve as powerful allies in the energetic transformation of any space, promoting balance, well-being, and protection for everyone who inhabits it.

30: Chakra Harmonization

Harmonizing the chakras with Arcturian crystals helps remove energetic blockages and restore the flow of vital energy. When the chakras are aligned, there is a balance between the physical, emotional, mental, and spiritual bodies, promoting overall well-being.

To harmonize your own chakras, the first step is to select the crystals that correspond to each energy center. Arcturian crystals have specific vibrations that resonate with each chakra, promoting balance and alignment. The crown chakra, located at the top of the head, is activated by the Violet Arcturian Crystal, whose vibrant color aids in spiritual connection. The third eye, between the eyebrows, benefits from the Indigo Blue Arcturian Crystal, enhancing intuition and mental clarity. For the throat chakra, situated at the base of the neck, the Light Blue Arcturian Crystal is used, fostering communication and authentic expression. At the center of the chest, the heart chakra can be balanced with either the Green Arcturian Crystal, which stimulates healing and unconditional love, or the Pink Arcturian Crystal, which strengthens feelings of compassion and warmth. The solar plexus, positioned above the navel, finds harmony with the Golden Arcturian Crystal, radiating personal power and confidence. The sacral chakra, located below the navel, resonates with the Orange Arcturian Crystal, stimulating creativity and vitality. Finally, the root chakra, at the base of the spine, is strengthened by the Red Arcturian Crystal, providing grounding and stability.

After selecting the appropriate crystals, it is essential to purify and energize them before use. Cleansing can be done using different methods, such as rinsing them under running water, smudging with herbs like sage or palo santo, or exposing them to sunlight or moonlight. During this process, it is important to hold each crystal and mentally set the intention for chakra alignment, amplifying its energy for harmonization.

Preparing for the harmonization session is a fundamental step. Choose a quiet environment where you will not be disturbed. Lie on your back on a comfortable surface and relax deeply, breathing slowly and mindfully to calm your mind and prepare your body to receive the energy.

With your body relaxed, place the crystals directly on their corresponding chakras. Close your eyes and visualize each chakra radiating its specific color, spinning freely and expanding its energy. This visualization helps enhance the effect of the crystals, allowing their vibration to integrate with your body's energy flow.

To activate the crystals' energy, focus on your breath and imagine a bright white light flowing through your body, cleansing and aligning each chakra. Remain in this position for 15 to 20 minutes, allowing the crystals to restore energetic balance.

At the end of the practice, slowly remove the crystals, starting from the root chakra and moving up to the crown chakra. Mentally express gratitude for the harmonization process, and to help integrate the energy into your physical body, drink a glass of water. This final step helps anchor the new vibrational frequency and promotes a lasting sense of well-being.

If the intention is to harmonize someone else's chakras, the process should be adapted to ensure they receive the crystal energy effectively. Begin by preparing the environment, choosing a peaceful location with soft lighting and, if possible, playing relaxing background music to encourage a state of serenity. Ask the person to lie on their back and relax, breathing deeply to calm the mind.

As with self-application, choose the appropriate crystals for the person's chakras and purify them before use. Cleansing and energizing the crystals are fundamental steps to ensure they are ready to work effectively in the harmonization process.

Once the crystals are prepared, place them on the corresponding chakras of the person's body. If necessary, adjust their positions to ensure proper alignment. Guide them to maintain steady, deep breaths, allowing the crystal energy to flow naturally.

To activate the energetic harmonization, use a selenite or white quartz wand, gently moving it over the crystals in a continuous flow, connecting them energetically. While doing this, visualize a bright light moving through the person's chakras, dissolving blockages and restoring a healthy energy flow.

After approximately 15 to 20 minutes, begin the closing process. Remove the crystals in the correct order, from the root chakra to the crown, allowing the energy to stabilize gradually. Ask the person to slowly open their eyes and share their sensations. Recommend that they drink a glass of water and rest for a few minutes to better absorb the harmonization effects.

To maintain balanced chakras in daily life, some practices can be incorporated into a routine. Whenever signs of imbalance arise, repeat this harmonization technique to restore energy flow. Meditating with a specific crystal on the corresponding chakra is also an excellent way to reinforce alignment. Additionally, wearing accessories such as necklaces or bracelets with Arcturian crystals can help maintain a stable vibration throughout the day.

By integrating this practice into your life, Arcturian crystals become powerful allies in energetic balance, promoting a deep sense of lightness, well-being, and overall harmony.

When selecting your Arcturian crystals, trust your intuition. Feel the crystal's energy and choose the one that resonates with you and your needs.

To care for your crystals, cleanse them regularly with running water, expose them to sunlight or moonlight to recharge, and store them in a safe, protected place.

Integrating Arcturian crystals into your healing journey opens the door to profound transformation and reconnection with your true essence. Each crystal carries a unique frequency, ready to assist in your process of balance and evolution. When used with intention and respect, they amplify their healing capabilities, creating a continuous flow of energy that harmonizes mind, body, and spirit. This subtle connection with the crystals transcends their physical use and expands into an energetic dialogue, where attuning to their vibrations reveals new paths of healing and self-discovery.

The relationship with Arcturian crystals also teaches the importance of care and reciprocity. Just as they provide energetic support, it is essential to keep them cleansed and energetically renewed. This constant care strengthens the bond between you and the crystal, making the interaction more fluid and effective. Over time, this practice becomes part of a sacred ritual, where each act of attention and gratitude reverberates through your energetic field, intensifying the energy exchange and deepening your spiritual connection.

Allow yourself to explore the wisdom contained in each crystal, recognizing them as allies in your multidimensional healing journey. Whether through meditation, crystal grids, or simple moments of contemplation, Arcturian crystals can serve as silent guides, awakening within you the remembrance of your true power and purpose. Thus, with love and intention, each crystal becomes a bridge between the earthly and the divine, leading you to higher states of consciousness and complete well-being.

Part 3

31: Sacred Geometry

The Arcturians possess profound knowledge of the vibrational structure of the universe, understanding that everything in existence is governed by mathematical patterns and geometric shapes that express the essence of creation. For them, Sacred Geometry is not merely an abstract concept but an active tool for interacting with cosmic forces, balancing energetic frequencies, and accessing higher dimensions of existence. Each shape, proportion, and numerical sequence carries a specific vibrational signature capable of influencing matter and consciousness. Through this understanding, the Arcturians employ Sacred Geometry to harmonize environments, facilitate spiritual ascension processes, and restore the energetic integrity of beings and planetary systems.

The interconnection between Sacred Geometry and the manifestation of reality is one of the fundamental principles governing their practices. They understand that by manipulating specific geometric patterns, they can reorganize the underlying energetic structure of any aspect of existence. In their ships and ethereal temples, they use shapes such as Metatron's Cube, the Flower of Life, and the Merkaba to stabilize frequencies and create fields of high vibrational resonance. These patterns not only serve as matrices of creation but also function as interdimensional portals, allowing consciousness to transition between different planes of reality. Thus, Sacred Geometry becomes a key to understanding the universal fabric and aligning with cosmic laws.

Ancient civilizations such as the Egyptians, Greeks, and Mayans intuitively grasped fragments of this knowledge and incorporated it into their architecture and sacred rituals. However, the Arcturians, with their advanced wisdom, have developed this science even further, revealing the hidden codes that permeate creation. From their perspective, Sacred Geometry not only reflects the order of the cosmos but also enables profound transformations at the cellular and spiritual levels. By applying these principles in their healing technologies, they can reconfigure imbalanced energetic structures, restoring original patterns of harmony and alignment. Their mastery of this universal language makes them experts in using form, light, and vibration to promote balance on all levels of existence.

To the Arcturians, each geometric shape possesses a specific vibration and purpose within the universal structure. The circle, for example, symbolizes unity and wholeness, while the triangle represents the fundamental triad of creation, such as body, mind, and spirit. The cube, in turn, manifests stability and the materialization of energy in the physical plane. These shapes are not merely symbolic representations but active tools that, when properly applied, can alter energetic patterns, open dimensional portals, and promote spiritual ascension.

The Arcturians apply this science in various fields, from the architecture of their ships and ethereal temples to the healing technologies they develop. Their structures are built based on highly resonant geometric patterns, ensuring that spaces maintain an elevated frequency and facilitate the expansion of consciousness. Their healing chambers, for instance, are designed using the Flower of Life, a geometric matrix that contains the fundamental sequence of creation. Within these chambers, the Arcturians utilize light, sound, and geometric shapes to restore harmony to subtle bodies, promoting deep healing on both physical and spiritual levels.

Furthermore, Sacred Geometry is also applied in the processes of Merkaba activation, the energetic field of light that surrounds each being and enables access to higher states of consciousness. The Merkaba, represented by two interlocked tetrahedrons, symbolizes the union of masculine and feminine energies and the interconnection between the material and spiritual worlds. When properly activated, it allows for interdimensional travel and facilitates alignment with the cosmic flows of creation. The Arcturians teach that activating this field of light is not merely a mental exercise but a process involving vibrational alignment, pure intention, and connection with the higher frequencies of the universe.

Another fundamental aspect of the Arcturians' use of Sacred Geometry is related to environmental and planetary harmonization. They understand that planetary energy fields also respond to geometric patterns, and thus, they use this science to stabilize frequencies and assist in collective evolution. During planetary transition periods, they project light mandalas based on Sacred Geometry to restore energetic balance and facilitate resonance with higher frequencies. These mandalas are not just symbolic drawings but vibrational structures that act directly upon Earth's subtle fields, promoting essential energetic recalibration for the ascension process.

The practical application of this knowledge can also be incorporated into daily human life. The Arcturians teach that meditating with geometric shapes can amplify spiritual connection and rebalance personal energy. One of the most commonly used methods is visualizing the Flower of Life around the body, imagining it pulsing with golden light and radiating harmony to all cells. Another powerful exercise is mentally constructing a dodecahedron around the energetic field, allowing its refined vibration to elevate personal frequency and support states of expanded consciousness.

Thus, Sacred Geometry is not just an abstract concept but a living tool that, when understood and correctly applied, enables a direct connection with the fundamental structure of the universe. With their deep understanding of this science, the Arcturians use it to create realities, harmonize dimensions, and expand consciousness beyond the limits of ordinary perception. Their knowledge invites us to rediscover this universal language and use it as a means of personal and collective transformation, awakening the remembrance of our own divine nature and the orderly flow that permeates all of creation.

Principles of Sacred Geometry

32: Unity

The interconnection between all forms of existence is sublimely manifested in Sacred Geometry, an ancient knowledge that reveals the fundamental patterns of creation. Every geometric structure present in nature, from snowflakes to galactic spirals, expresses the underlying harmony of the universe, reflecting the essential unity that permeates all existence. Understanding this deep connection allows the mind to transcend the illusion of separation, recognizing that everything is part of a vast energetic fabric. This recognition is not merely theoretical but experiential, providing an expansion of consciousness that transcends the limitations of everyday perception. Thus, delving into Sacred Geometry is not just about contemplating shapes but directly experiencing the interconnectedness of the cosmos and the presence of unity in all things.

The energetic harmonization through Sacred Geometry occurs through the resonance between universal patterns and the internal structure of each being. Just as the body's cells follow a precise design aligned with the golden proportions and fundamental geometric shapes, the human energy field responds to the presence of sacred symbols, amplifying its vibration and attuning to higher frequencies. By interacting with patterns such as the Flower of Life, the Merkaba, and Metatron's Cube, a natural alignment occurs, facilitating connection with the cosmic flow and stimulating spiritual awakening. This energetic interaction is not limited to the individual sphere but reverberates through all aspects of existence, promoting balance, mental clarity, and a profound sense of belonging to the whole. By integrating this wisdom into daily life, it is possible to transform not only the perception of reality but also the very experience of life, making it more fluid, harmonious, and conscious.

The practice of Sacred Geometry as a tool for spiritual elevation involves both the contemplation of these patterns and immersion in the vibration they emit. Creating a space dedicated to connecting with these geometric forms allows the environment to become an energetic portal to expanded states of consciousness. Placing sacred symbols in strategic locations, meditating while visualizing geometric structures, or simply observing the perfect symmetry present in nature are ways to attune to this universal language. When the mind opens to this perception, a profound internal realignment occurs, dissolving energetic blockages and expanding consciousness beyond the boundaries of the individual self. Thus, Sacred Geometry not only reveals the unity of creation but also becomes a means of fully experiencing it, allowing each human being to recognize their innate connection with the infinite.

To embark on this journey toward Unity through Sacred Geometry, it is essential to prepare the environment appropriately, creating a space conducive to energetic and spiritual connection. Choose a quiet place where you will not be interrupted, ensuring that your full attention is focused on the process. To enhance the energy of the space, light a candle or use incense of your choice, allowing the aroma and soft flame to elevate the surrounding vibration. Additionally, place sacred symbols such as the Flower of Life, the Merkaba, or Metatron's Cube in strategic points within the space. These symbols contain geometric patterns that resonate with the structure of the universe, aiding in energetic harmonization and facilitating connection with the whole.

Once the environment is properly prepared, the next step is aligning your intention. Sit comfortably with your spine straight and take a few deep breaths. Allow each inhale and exhale to relax your body and calm your mind. Then, close your eyes and visualize a golden field of energy surrounding you. Feel this energy filling every cell of your body and gradually expanding, connecting you to the Creative Source. Mentally set your intention to integrate with the cosmic unity, recognizing that you, all living beings, and the entire universe are part of a single energetic flow. The clearer this intention, the deeper the effect of this practice will be.

Now, enter the meditation phase of connection. Focus on the center of your chest and visualize a sphere of white light gently pulsating in your heart. Imagine this light growing and radiating beyond your body, enveloping everything around you. Gradually, this light expands even further, reaching all people, living beings, and even the Earth itself. Allow yourself to dissolve into this light, feeling that there is no separation between you and the universe. You are the whole, and the whole is you. Remain in this state of contemplation and connection for at least ten minutes, allowing your consciousness to expand and perceive this deep interconnection.

If you wish to share this experience and help someone else feel this unity, guide them through this process carefully. Explain each step and encourage them to follow the same process, ensuring that they are comfortable and receptive. If you notice any difficulty, assist them through a guided meditation, narrating each part of the connection process with the whole. To enhance the experience, use Sacred Geometry symbols near the person's energy field. You can mentally or physically project the image of the Flower of Life or Metatron's Cube over them, facilitating the perception of unity and strengthening their spiritual connection.

After the meditation, it is essential to anchor the experience and conclude the process consciously. Ask the person to take a few deep breaths, bringing their awareness back to their physical body and the present moment. Reinforce the experience by encouraging them to express in words how they felt during the process. Verbalizing the experience helps make it more concrete and integrated into consciousness. Conclude the process with a gesture of gratitude, thanking the Creative Source and the energetic field itself for the opportunity for connection and alignment.

The benefits of this practice are numerous and profound. The expansion of consciousness and the perception of the whole become increasingly present in daily life, bringing a new perspective on reality and the self. Spiritual connection is strengthened, providing a sense of belonging and harmony. Additionally, the practice helps reduce feelings of separation and isolation, promoting a sense of unity and unconditional love. Finally, vibrational frequency is elevated, allowing for a state of greater balance and alignment with universal energies.

33: Patterns

The structure of the universe reveals geometric patterns that repeat from the smallest particles to vast galaxies, expressing a cosmic order that permeates all existence. Sacred Geometry, by manifesting these primordial forms, not only reflects the harmony of the universe but also acts as a powerful tool for energetic connection and consciousness expansion. These patterns, such as the Golden Spiral, the Flower of Life, and Metatron's Cube, represent the fundamental organization of matter and energy, becoming keys to understanding the interconnectedness between the human being and the whole. By observing and interacting with these geometric forms, the mind naturally aligns with higher frequencies, facilitating processes of balance, spiritual activation, and healing. This attunement is not merely visual or intellectual but vibrational, directly influencing the energetic structure of each individual and allowing a reconnection with the harmonic flow of creation.

The conscious use of Sacred Geometry in energetic harmonization involves both the contemplation of these patterns and their practical application in environments and meditative processes. Creating a space where these forms are present—

whether through images, objects, or visualizations—helps elevate the vibration of the place and intensifies alignment with universal forces. When a sacred symbol like the Flower of Life is present, for example, it resonates with the same patterns that structure nature and the human body, promoting balance and stability. Similarly, the Golden Spiral, reflected in natural phenomena such as seashells and galaxies, inspires expansion and inner growth. Working with these geometric forms allows access to expanded states of perception, dissolving energetic blockages and facilitating alignment with higher frequencies. This practice, in addition to restoring internal balance, broadens awareness of the presence of these patterns in all manifestations of reality, strengthening the connection between the individual and the universe.

Incorporating Sacred Geometry into a spiritual routine provides a journey of self-knowledge and integration with cosmic laws. Meditating with these forms, visualizing their presence in the energy body, or applying them in therapeutic practices are ways to anchor their energy in daily life. As perception expands, it becomes easier to recognize the underlying unity of all things, dissolving the illusion of separation and fostering a state of deep connection with universal intelligence. By understanding that the same patterns that organize galaxies also structure human biology, a new perspective on life and the self emerges, bringing greater clarity, harmony, and balance. In this way, Sacred Geometry not only reveals itself as valuable ancient knowledge but also as a practical path for raising personal vibration and attuning to the perfect order of the universe.

To begin this practice of energetic harmonization through Sacred Geometry, it is essential to create an environment conducive to connection and the perception of universal patterns. Choose a quiet, clean, and organized place where you feel comfortable and free from distractions. To enhance the experience, use images or objects that represent sacred geometric patterns, such as mandalas, crystals engraved with the Flower of Life, or representations of Metatron's Cube. These elements help anchor energy and intensify alignment with cosmic order. Lighting a candle or incense can contribute to creating an atmosphere of serenity and introspection, fostering a deeper connection with the subtle patterns that govern existence.

With the space prepared, close your eyes and take deep breaths, allowing yourself to relax and enter a state of mindfulness. Focus on how geometric patterns manifest in nature and how they are present in different scales of reality. Imagine the golden spiral appearing in seashells, in distant galaxies, and in whirlwinds formed by the wind. Visualize the perfect hexagons of honeycombs, structured with precision and efficiency. Bring to mind the Flower of Life, a pattern found in cells and plant growth forms, reflecting the harmony that permeates all existence. As you observe these patterns, notice how everything follows an ordered and perfect flow, revealing the presence of a universal intelligence governing creation.

Now, choose one of the geometric patterns to work with energetically. It could be the Flower of Life, symbolizing interconnectedness; the Golden Spiral, representing infinite growth and expansion; or Metatron's Cube, associated with spiritual activation and energetic harmony. Visualize this pattern forming above you as a luminous and vibrant grid. Feel this geometric structure gently descending, enveloping your body and aligning your energy field. Allow this energy to flow through every cell of your being, dissolving blockages, balancing emotions, and bringing mental clarity. With each breath, imagine this geometric light pulsing in sync with your heart, expanding and strengthening your connection with the universe. Remain in this state of integration for at least ten minutes, absorbing the benefits of the experience.

If you wish to apply this practice to another person, invite them to lie down in a comfortable position, preferably in a quiet place. Hold an image or an object representing the chosen geometric pattern near their energy field. Guide them to breathe deeply and relax, preparing to receive the harmonization. Begin by leading a visualization: describe how a luminous geometric pattern forms around their body, enveloping them in restorative energy. Explain that this luminous structure is balancing their energies, removing blockages, and promoting a state of deep harmony. You can enhance the process by using directed affirmations, such as: "The energy of the Flower of Life is restoring your inner harmony" or "Metatron's Cube is activating your higher consciousness." If you feel it is appropriate, gently trace the patterns in the air above the person's body, as if drawing their invisible forms with your hands, intensifying the connection and energetic activation.

To conclude the practice, ask the person to take a few deep breaths and bring their awareness back to the present moment. Encourage them to share their sensations and experiences during the process, allowing them to verbalize what they perceived. Guide them to maintain awareness of geometric patterns in daily life, observing how they manifest in different forms around them. This exercise will expand their perception of universal harmony, reinforcing their connection with the natural flow of creation and promoting a continuous state of balance and well-being.

By incorporating this practice into your routine, you can experience significant benefits, such as a greater awareness of universal order and harmony, deeper energetic and emotional balance, and an expansion of consciousness through Sacred Geometry. Additionally, the sense of connection with the natural flow of life will become more present, providing a journey of self-discovery and alignment with the universe.

34: Golden Ratio

The Golden Ratio, represented by the number Phi (≈1.618), is a mathematical manifestation of the harmony present throughout creation. From the structure of the human body to the organization of galaxies, this ratio governs the way nature expresses itself, reflecting an intrinsic balance that resonates with the fundamental principles of existence. Its presence can be observed in plant growth, the arrangement of sunflower seeds, the spiral of seashells, and even in the anatomy of living beings. This universal pattern is not merely an aesthetic construct but also a reflection of cosmic intelligence, organizing matter and energy in a way that favors the natural flow of life. When applied consciously, the Golden Ratio becomes a powerful tool for energetic realignment, consciousness elevation, and harmonization with the natural rhythms of the universe.

Attunement to this frequency can be cultivated through the observation and interaction with geometric forms that follow this proportion, awakening a deep connection between the human being and cosmic order. Simply contemplating Golden Ratio patterns in nature already has a vibrational impact, stimulating a state of inner balance. To enhance this experience, it is possible to integrate the Golden Ratio into meditative and energetic practices, using objects such as mandalas, pyramids, and golden spirals to anchor this vibration in the subtle field. By consciously visualizing these patterns, the mind aligns with universal harmony, allowing for a more balanced energy flow and an expanded perception of the interconnectedness of all things. This practice not only promotes relaxation and mental clarity but also acts as a catalyst for consciousness expansion, facilitating access to higher states of perception and understanding.

Incorporating the Golden Ratio into the spiritual journey is a continuous process that is reflected both in external contemplation and internal alignment. Meditation with the Golden Spiral, for example, strengthens the connection with this universal structure, stimulating attunement with the natural rhythms of existence. By visualizing this spiral expanding from the center of the chest and enveloping the entire body, a resonance field is created with primordial harmony, dissolving energetic blockages and promoting a state of deep integration. Likewise, applying these principles to the environment, art, architecture, and even body movement helps reconnect with the geometry of life. This awareness transforms how reality is perceived, allowing the order and beauty of the universe to become a tangible and present experience in daily life. By cultivating this connection, each human being can realign their vibration with the cosmic flow and experience a continuous state of harmony and well-being.

To begin this practice of connection with the Golden Ratio, it is essential to properly prepare the space. Choose a quiet environment where you feel comfortable and free from interruptions. This space should convey harmony and serenity, facilitating immersion in the exercise. To intensify attunement with the energy of the Golden Ratio, use objects that embody this proportion in their natural structure, such as seashells, mandalas, pyramids, or images of the Golden Spiral. These elements serve as visual and vibrational anchors, reinforcing the connection with this frequency. Additionally, lighting a candle or placing crystals in the environment can enhance the energetic vibration, creating a field conducive to the practice.

Once the space is prepared, sit comfortably and begin connecting with natural harmony. Take several deep breaths, inhaling slowly through the nose and exhaling gently through the mouth, allowing each breath to calm your mind and relax your body. Direct your attention to a natural element that contains the Golden Ratio—it could be a flower, a seashell, or even an image of a spiral galaxy. If no physical object is available, mentally visualize one of these forms. Observe how this structure manifests in nature spontaneously and perfectly, reflecting balance and beauty in all things. As you observe, allow yourself to feel this harmony resonating within you, bringing a deep sense of alignment with the natural flow of existence.

Now, with a serene mind connected to the energy of the Golden Ratio, move on to energetic activation with the Golden Spiral. Close your eyes and gently visualize this spiral beginning to form at the center of your chest, exactly at the heart chakra. Imagine it spinning harmoniously, gradually expanding and radiating a golden light that envelops your entire being. Feel this energy flowing smoothly through your body, restoring your energetic balance and promoting a deep sense of harmony. Remain in this state, breathing consciously and allowing this spiral to align your vibration with the natural order of the universe. To maximize the experience, stay with this visualization for at least ten minutes, allowing the energy to stabilize and integrate into your energy field.

If you wish to apply this technique to another person, follow a similar process, ensuring they are also comfortable and relaxed. Ask them to lie down in a position that promotes relaxation and deep breathing. Guide them to inhale and exhale slowly, releasing any accumulated tension. Then, with gentle hand movements, trace the Golden Spiral in the air above their body, starting from the center of their chest and expanding outward. Visualize the energy of this spiral completely surrounding them, restoring their harmony and energetic balance. To intensify the process, you can use a crystal carved into the shape of the Golden Spiral or place objects that follow the Golden Ratio near their body, allowing these vibrations to act on their energy field.

After completing the practice, it is essential to anchor and conclude the process. Ask the person to take a few deep breaths, bringing their awareness back to the present moment. Encourage them to share their perceptions and sensations during the experience, promoting a conscious integration of what was felt. Additionally, suggest that they observe the Golden Ratio in nature and even in the forms of their own body, developing a deeper awareness of universal harmony.

The benefits of this practice are vast and include the restoration of energetic balance, alignment with natural harmony, an expanded awareness of universal patterns, and a profound sense of peace and fulfillment. By incorporating this technique into daily life, it is possible to strengthen the connection with the energy of the universe and experience a continuous state of well-being and harmony.

35: Vibration

Vibration is the primordial essence that permeates all existence, connecting every form and structure to universal harmony. Everything in the universe, from atoms to galaxies, emits specific vibrational frequencies, influencing the energy of living beings and the surrounding environment. In Sacred Geometry, these vibrations manifest through forms and patterns that resonate with the fundamental structure of the cosmos. The Arcturians, beings known for their elevated consciousness and advanced knowledge of subtle energies, use these vibrations to promote healing, balance, and spiritual expansion. Understanding and consciously working with this energy enables profound vibrational adjustments, allowing for the elevation of personal frequency and the harmonization of the energetic field. When we attune our own vibrations to high-frequency geometric patterns, we open a channel for a purer energy flow aligned with universal laws.

The practical application of this knowledge involves the intentional use of geometric shapes, sound, and visualization to create a state of harmonic resonance in the body and mind. Each geometric symbol carries a unique vibrational signature, capable of interacting with energy centers and subtly adjusting the flow of vital energy. The Merkaba, for example, acts as a field of protection and spiritual activation, while the Flower of Life aids in energetic balance and alignment with universal patterns of creation. Metatron's Cube intensifies the connection with higher dimensions, facilitating consciousness expansion and vibrational elevation. When combined with specific sound frequencies, such as sacred mantras, Solfeggio frequencies, or binaural beats, these geometric patterns become even more powerful, amplifying their effects on the individual energy field. This interaction between form and sound creates a resonance field that can be directed toward healing, spiritual alignment, and the activation of expanded states of perception.

By integrating this practice into daily life, one develops a heightened sensitivity to the vibration of forms and sounds, allowing for a deeper attunement to the subtle frequencies that govern existence. Visualizing sacred geometries, combined with the conscious emission of harmonic sounds, strengthens the auric field and balances the chakras, restoring energetic fluidity and promoting a state of inner peace. Additionally, connecting with these vibrations facilitates spiritual awakening, providing a broader understanding of the interconnectedness of all things. Incorporating this knowledge into a routine—whether through meditation, the use of symbols in the environment, or listening to specific sound frequencies—enables continuous vibrational transformation, aligning the self with the highest frequencies of creation. Thus, the vibration of Sacred Geometry becomes not just a concept to be studied but a lived experience capable of expanding consciousness and strengthening the connection with the universal energy flow.

Before beginning the practice, it is essential to prepare the environment to ensure that energy flows freely and is enhanced. Choose a quiet space where there will be no interruptions, and if possible, harmonize it using elements that resonate with Sacred Geometry. Position specific crystals or objects representing high-vibration geometric forms, such as Metatron's Cube, the Merkaba, or the Flower of Life. These symbols help amplify the energy of the space, creating a field conducive to the practice. To intensify the experience, you can add high-frequency music, such as binaural beats, Solfeggio frequencies, or harmonic chants, as these sound vibrations assist in attunement with subtle planes.

Once the environment is properly prepared, sit comfortably and begin a process of deep, conscious breathing. Inhale slowly, filling your lungs, and exhale gently, releasing any tension or energetic blockages. As your mind calms, start visualizing luminous geometric shapes around you, vibrating at different frequencies. Feel these geometries pulsating in harmony with your energy, expanding and filling the entire space with their light. Choose a specific geometry to work with—the Merkaba for protection, the Flower of Life for balance, or Metatron's Cube for spiritual elevation. Allow this geometric form to integrate into your energy field, absorbing its vibration and adjusting your internal frequency.

Now, introduce sound vibration to intensify this connection. Choose a vocal sound that resonates with you, such as the sacred "OM," and chant it softly while maintaining the visualization of the sacred geometry. If preferred, use vibrational instruments such as Tibetan singing bowls, bells, or tuning forks to amplify the effects of the practice. As the sound reverberates, observe how it interacts with the chosen geometric form, enhancing its energy and creating a harmonic resonance within and around you. Feel this vibration expanding through your body, aligning your energy centers and promoting a profound state of balance and connection.

If you wish to apply this technique to another person, ask them to lie down comfortably and relax. Choose the geometric form most suitable for their energy field and visualize it pulsing with light and energy above them. With your hands, trace the geometry in the air over their body, directing the vibration with the intention of healing and harmonization. If using sound, position yourself near the chakra that needs adjustment and emit the corresponding vibration, allowing the resonance to act directly on energy restoration. During the process, reinforce your intention with positive affirmations, such as: "Feel the vibration of Sacred Geometry restoring your energy and elevating your consciousness." Observe the person's reactions, respecting their time and perceptions.

To conclude the practice, it is essential to anchor the energies worked with and bring awareness back to a normal state. Ask the person to take a few deep breaths, feeling present in the here and now. Discuss the sensations experienced and offer guidance on how they can continue connecting with geometric vibrations in their daily life. Suggest practices such as frequent visualization of these forms, listening to harmonic sounds, or physically engaging with geometric symbols in objects and artifacts.

By integrating this practice into daily life, the benefits become evident: vibrational frequency elevation, deep energetic harmonization, expanded consciousness, and the activation of elevated meditative states. Sacred Geometry is a powerful tool for transformation and alignment, allowing the connection with the universal energy field to become increasingly fluid and natural.

36: Symbols

The symbols of Sacred Geometry carry vibrational patterns capable of influencing the energy of the environment and individuals who come into contact with them. Present in various cultures and spiritual traditions, these geometric forms are not merely visual representations but portals of connection to higher dimensions and subtle energy fields. The Flower of Life, the Merkaba, the Tree of Life, and Metatron's Cube are some of the most powerful examples, each playing specific roles in harmonization, protection, and consciousness elevation. Used for millennia by ancient civilizations, these symbols remain relevant today, applied in meditative practices, energy therapies, and studies on the fundamental structure of the universe. Their impact goes beyond aesthetics or esoteric knowledge; they represent the universal language of creation, encoding mathematical and spiritual principles that govern reality.

Interacting with these symbols can be deeply transformative when done with intention and understanding. The first step in accessing their frequencies is to establish a suitable space for this connection. A harmonized environment not only facilitates alignment with the symbols but also amplifies the effects of their subtle energies. Elements such as crystals, mandalas, and incense help elevate vibrational frequencies, creating an energetic field that facilitates contact with higher dimensions. Additionally, choosing the appropriate symbol for each situation is essential to maximize its benefits. Each geometric form carries a distinct energetic signature, influencing different aspects of the self and the environment. The Flower of Life, for example, resonates with cosmic harmony and unity, while the Merkaba acts as a vehicle for spiritual ascension and protection. Metatron's Cube, on the other hand, possesses strong purifying and energetic alignment power, functioning as a channel for transmuting dense energies. By understanding these properties, it becomes possible to use these symbols in a targeted manner, promoting balance and spiritual expansion.

The practical application of these symbols primarily occurs through meditation and visualization. By focusing on a specific symbol, whether by holding a physical representation or mentally projecting its image, an energetic resonance process begins. This practice allows for the absorption of the beneficial vibrations of sacred geometry, facilitating the harmonization of the auric field and the activation of latent consciousness potentials. During meditation, conscious breathing and clear intention intensify this connection, enabling expanded states of perception. For those who wish to go beyond individual experience, these symbols can be used in energy therapies to assist in restoring the vibrational balance of others. By placing a symbol over a specific energy center of the body or tracing its shape in the air, a healing field is created that directly acts on a person's frequency, alleviating blockages and strengthening vital energy. Integrating these symbols into daily life—whether through amulets, sacred art, or regular spiritual practices—helps maintain a continuous state of alignment and energetic protection, fostering a journey of self-knowledge and connection with the divine.

To deeply connect with the symbols of Sacred Geometry and access their powerful energetic frequencies, it is essential to follow a structured process involving preparation, conscious symbol selection, meditation, and application on oneself or others. Each step strengthens alignment with these subtle energies, allowing for a more intense and transformative experience.

The first step is preparing the space, as an appropriate environment enhances energetic connection and intensifies the effects of the practice. Choose a quiet place free from interruptions and harmonize it in a way that reflects peace and serenity. Position sacred geometric symbols around, such as mandalas, engraved crystals, or representations of the Flower of Life, the Merkaba, or Metatron's Cube. These elements serve as energetic anchors, helping to establish a high-frequency field in the environment. To further enhance this atmosphere, light a candle or incense of your choice, allowing the aromas to aid in vibrational elevation and the creation of a conducive spiritual connection field.

With the space properly prepared, the next step involves selecting the appropriate symbol. Each figure in Sacred Geometry has a specific vibration and influences different aspects of personal and environmental energy. If the goal is balance and harmony, the Flower of Life is the best choice, as its structure represents the interconnectedness of all existence. For those seeking energetic protection and spiritual activation, the Merkaba stands out, as it symbolizes a light vehicle capable of expanding consciousness. The Tree of Life is ideal for deepening spiritual connection and understanding life cycles. If the need is energy cleansing and vibrational elevation, Metatron's Cube fulfills this role, as it contains all geometric shapes that structure creation, acting as a powerful purifier of dense energies.

After selecting the most suitable symbol, meditation with the symbol begins—this is the moment of immersion and attunement with its frequency. Sit comfortably, preferably in a quiet place, and hold the chosen symbol or visualize it clearly. Close your eyes and take deep breaths, allowing your mind to calm and your subtle perception to expand. Imagine the symbol shining intensely and, as you breathe, visualize this light expanding around you, forming a protective and harmonizing energy field. Let yourself be enveloped by this energy, allowing it to fill every cell of your body, balancing your vibration. Remain in this meditative state for approximately 10 to 15 minutes, or as long as you feel necessary, absorbing the qualities and strength of the symbol into your energetic field.

If you wish to expand this practice to help others, you can apply the technique of using symbols for the energetic harmonization of third parties. To do this, ask the person to lie down comfortably, allowing them to enter a state of deep relaxation. Choose a symbol according to their need and place it near the corresponding chakra. For example, if the intention is spiritual expansion, the Merkaba can be placed over the heart chakra, facilitating openness to higher frequencies. When positioning the symbol, visualize its energy gently flowing into the person's body, restoring their vibrational balance and dissolving energetic blockages. If preferred, you can also draw the symbol in the air with your hands, tracing its shape while projecting intentions of healing, harmony, and protection. To enhance the effects, use powerful affirmations, such as: "The energy of the Flower of Life restores your balance and connection with the divine." These words function as vibrational commands that reinforce the integration of the symbol's energy into the person's subtle field.

Finally, the closing and integration stage is reached, where the transition from the meditative experience to a normal state of consciousness should occur smoothly. After the practice, ask the person to take a few deep breaths, slowly returning to awareness of their surroundings. Ask about their sensations and experiences, allowing them to express how they felt during the process. To maintain the benefits throughout the day, recommend that they carry a small representation of the symbol used, whether as a pendant, drawing, or engraved crystal. This will help keep their vibration elevated and maintain a connection with the energy worked on in the practice.

The benefits of this process are numerous. Connecting with Sacred Geometry symbols strengthens spirituality, promotes deep energetic harmonization, and creates a protective layer against negative external influences. Additionally, it facilitates the expansion of consciousness, allowing access to elevated states of meditation and perception. By incorporating these practices into daily life, it is possible to experience continuous inner transformation, aligning more and more with universal energies and awakening a state of balance and fulfillment.

37: Healing Codes of Sacred Geometry

The Healing Codes of Sacred Geometry represent a bridge between universal laws and human experience, carrying a vibration capable of restoring energetic balance on multiple levels. These geometric patterns, infused with ancestral knowledge and cosmic intelligence, function as tools for reconfiguring the energetic matrix, dissolving blockages, and realigning frequencies to promote the integral harmony of the being. By interacting with these sacred forms—whether through visualization, mental projection, or inscription on physical surfaces—one accesses a vibrational field of information that transcends the limits of time and space, activating profound and transformative healing processes. Their application is not limited to the physical body but extends to emotional, mental, and spiritual levels, fostering systemic restoration that supports both the expansion of consciousness and the strengthening of the connection with higher dimensions.

Each geometric code carries a specific energetic signature, resonating with distinct aspects of existence and serving as a channel for manifesting cosmic order in material reality. The activation of these codes occurs when the mind and conscious intention align with the frequency they represent, allowing their vibration to integrate into the auric field and initiate a resonance process. This phenomenon can be observed in both individual practices and collective energy therapies, where the codes are used to restore the flow of vital energy, unblock repressed emotions, and realign energy centers. The use of crystals, sounds, and mantras enhances this interaction, amplifying the effects and creating a field of harmony that extends beyond the individual, also influencing the surrounding environment.

Among the most commonly used symbols in this context are Metatron's Cube, the Flower of Life, and the Merkaba, each playing an essential role in the process of healing and spiritual ascension. Metatron's Cube is a powerful channel for protection and alignment, capable of dissolving dense energies and strengthening the vibrational field. The Flower of Life, in turn, contains the fundamental patterns of creation, promoting the restoration of inner harmony and the activation of the being's latent potential. The Merkaba functions as an interdimensional light vehicle, facilitating deep spiritual connections and expanding consciousness beyond the limitations of the three-dimensional reality. Integrating these codes into daily life allows for a constant realignment with the forces that sustain universal order, fostering balance, protection, and continuous evolution. By engaging with the Healing Codes of Sacred Geometry, one opens a path to self-knowledge and inner transformation, enabling the original vibration of the soul to fully manifest in earthly existence.

These codes operate as energetic keys capable of unlocking limiting patterns, releasing stagnant energies, and realigning the subtle bodies, promoting healing and expanded awareness on multiple levels. They function as energetic catalysts that, when correctly applied, harmonize an individual's frequencies, eliminate emotional blockages, alleviate physical pain, restore energy flow, and strengthen the connection with higher dimensions. Their action is subtle yet profoundly transformative, as they directly influence the vibrational fields that structure reality and human experience.

Sacred Geometry contains the fundamental principles that govern the harmony of the universe, and through the Healing Codes, this cosmic mathematics can be used to reconfigure the body's energy, bringing it back to its natural state of balance and wholeness. There are different ways to apply these codes, each providing a unique experience of connection and transformation.

One of the most common methods of activation is visualization, in which one mentally imagines the sacred geometry vibrating and interacting with the energetic field, dissolving blockages and restoring the flow of vital energy. This technique can be enhanced by focusing on breathing and setting a specific intention for healing. Drawing the codes—whether in the air with the hands, on the skin, or on specific surfaces—helps anchor these frequencies on a more physical level, making the experience even more tangible.

Mental projection is another powerful technique, where one visualizes the geometry being integrated into their own body or environment, expanding its vibrational influence. This method can be used for personal healing as well as for harmonizing spaces and assisting others by projecting the codes directly into their energy fields. The use of crystals enhances this practice, as these stones can be programmed with healing codes and placed on chakras or specific points on the body to amplify their effect. Quartz, amethyst, and selenite are especially recommended for this type of work.

Another effective approach is the use of sounds and mantras, as sound vibrations resonate directly with sacred geometry, activating its healing properties. Each code has a specific frequency that can be amplified through vocal intonations, chants, or even musical instruments. Sounds like "OM" or binaural frequencies can be combined with the visualization of the codes to create an even more powerful vibrational field.

Among the Arcturian Healing Codes, some of the most well-known include Metatron's Cube, which promotes deep energetic realignment, clears blockages, and offers spiritual protection. The Flower of Life, a symbol of universal creation, is used to balance vital energies, restore emotional harmony, and elevate an individual's vibration. The Merkaba, in turn, activates the light body and facilitates connection with higher dimensions, promoting a profound expansion of consciousness.

The Golden Spiral of Fibonacci is another essential code, representing the continuous flow of vital energy and cellular regeneration, assisting in physical healing and reconnection with the natural order of the universe. The Tree of Life symbolizes the connection between spirit and matter, fostering deep alignment between the different aspects of the being. Each of these codes can be used individually or in combination, depending on the specific healing and transformation needs of the moment.

The practice of Arcturian Healing Codes is not limited to individual use; it can be applied to other people, environments, and even situations, helping to dissolve dense energies and restore harmony in various contexts. During a healing session, the practitioner can mentally project the codes onto the recipient's energy field, draw them with their hands, or use objects containing these sacred symbols to amplify their vibration.

The Arcturians teach that by resonating with these geometric forms, a transformation field opens, allowing a person to absorb higher energies and restructure their own vibrational frequency. This knowledge can be integrated into spiritual practices, holistic therapies, meditations, and self-transformation processes. By consciously connecting with the Healing Codes of Sacred Geometry, you access an energetic flow that transcends matter and aligns your essence with the universal field of creation, allowing healing and evolution to occur in a profound and lasting way.

38: Flower of Life

The Flower of Life manifests the fundamental structure of creation, revealing the mathematical and geometric perfection that sustains all existence. This sacred pattern, found in various cultures and traditions throughout history, is a visual expression of the interconnectedness of all life forms and the universal principles that govern reality. Composed of a sequence of symmetrically overlapping circles, the Flower of Life contains within its structure the secrets of cosmic harmony, reflecting the primordial language of the universe. Its geometry is directly linked to the process of matter formation, the organization of subatomic particles, and the flow of vital energy that permeates all planes of existence. Through it, one can access profound knowledge about creation, consciousness, and the interconnection between the physical and spiritual worlds.

The Arcturians, highly evolved beings in both consciousness and spiritual technology, use the Flower of Life as a tool for harmonization and energetic alignment. Its use goes beyond visual contemplation, extending into advanced practices of healing, meditation, and higher consciousness activation. The structure of the Flower of Life resonates with the frequency of the universe's primordial forms, allowing for the reorganization of the subtle energies that compose the human being. By interacting with this sacred geometric field, the chakras become balanced, the aura is purified, and misaligned vibrational patterns are restored to their original state of harmony and perfection. This process not only strengthens the individual's energy field but also facilitates connection with higher dimensions, expanding perception and awakening ancestral memories dormant within the spiritual DNA.

Beyond its influence on the energetic body, the Flower of Life is a key to accessing cosmic records and understanding the underlying structure of reality. It contains within itself all the geometric forms that underpin creation, including Metatron's Cube, the Platonic solids, and the Merkaba, representing the interaction between space, time, and consciousness. This universal matrix is used by the Arcturians to facilitate ascension processes, accelerate spiritual evolution, and integrate human beings into higher states of awareness. By meditating on this sacred pattern or working directly with its vibration, it is possible to unlock internal potentials, restore connection with universal wisdom, and attune to the true essence of the cosmos.

39: Merkaba

The Merkaba is a field of light that surrounds the human body, activating the Light Body and facilitating ascension. It consists of two tetrahedrons rotating in opposite directions, creating an energetic vortex that connects the individual to higher dimensions. The Arcturians use the Merkaba to promote multidimensional healing, consciousness expansion, and connection with the Higher Self.

To apply the Merkaba to oneself, it is essential to create a suitable environment and prepare both the body and mind for the activation of this powerful sacred geometry. The first step is to find a quiet place where you will not be interrupted, ensuring that the practice unfolds without distractions. Sitting comfortably with your spine straight and feet firmly on the ground, begin to breathe deeply, inhaling through your nose and exhaling slowly through your mouth. This conscious breathing helps to calm the mind and align your energy. Next, visualize a flow of golden light descending from the universe and gently entering through the top of your head, filling your entire being with a warm and purifying energy.

With the body and mind prepared, the next step is the activation of the sacred geometry of the Merkaba.

Imagine two interconnected tetrahedrons around you—one pointing upward and the other downward. The upper tetrahedron, representing masculine energy and spirit, begins to spin clockwise, while the lower one, symbolizing feminine energy and matter, spins counterclockwise. As these Platonic solids increase their rotational speed, a bright, pulsating field of light forms around you. Visualize this luminous field working on your energy, dissolving emotional blockages, balancing your chakras, and expanding your consciousness. Feel the subtle vibration of this sacred geometry harmonizing your being on a deep level.

As the rotation of the Merkaba intensifies, perceive your energy rising, transcending the limits of the physical body. Feel yourself expanding beyond the three-dimensional reality, connecting with higher planes of existence. Imagine this energetic structure aligning with the frequency of the Arcturians, allowing a direct flow of healing and universal wisdom. To reinforce this connection, mentally affirm: "I activate my Merkaba and allow my consciousness to expand in harmony and light." Remain in this elevated vibrational state for a few minutes, absorbing the subtle frequencies of sacred geometry.

After this transformative experience, it is crucial to ground the energy. Slowly visualize the rotation of the tetrahedrons gradually slowing down until they stabilize around your body. Feel your energy perfectly integrated and aligned, in balance with your essence. Take a deep breath, gently move your body, and when you feel ready, open your eyes. This careful conclusion ensures that the practice is completed in a balanced way, allowing the benefits of the Merkaba to be fully assimilated.

Just as it is possible to activate the Merkaba within oneself, this sacred geometry can also be applied to others to promote healing and consciousness expansion. The first step is to create an appropriate energetic space. Ask the person receiving the activation to lie down or sit comfortably, guiding them to breathe deeply and relax. Then, visualize a circle of light surrounding you both, creating a sacred field of protection and high vibration.

With the energetic space established, proceed to activate the Merkaba around the person. Place your hands over them—or, if preferred, visualize them surrounded by a field of radiant light. Imagine the two tetrahedrons spinning in opposite directions around their body, forming an energetic vortex that purifies and strengthens their spiritual structure. Visualize a golden light descending from the universe and completely enveloping them, activating their Light Body and elevating their vibration.

To deepen the experience, encourage the person to visualize or sense their energy rising, connecting with their Higher Self. This process can be intensified by repeating Arcturian mantras or affirmations that reinforce the connection with higher dimensions. Additionally, the use of harmonic sounds and frequencies such as 852 Hz and 963 Hz can be a powerful tool for facilitating spiritual activation, promoting elevated states of consciousness.

After activation, it is essential to close the process carefully. Gradually slow the rotation of the Merkaba, visualizing it stabilizing around the person. Guide them to move their body gently before standing up to ensure their energy is well-grounded. Finally, share insights or sensations that may have arisen during the practice, as these perceptions can provide valuable messages for the spiritual growth process.

The practice of the Merkaba offers numerous benefits, one of the most notable being the expansion of consciousness. By activating this sacred geometry, an individual experiences an enhanced perception, gaining access to new dimensions of wisdom and spiritual understanding. Additionally, the Merkaba significantly strengthens the energy field, functioning as a vibrational shield that protects against dense and unbalanced energies.

Another fundamental benefit is access to higher frequencies. This activation allows alignment with elevated planes of existence, facilitating communication with spiritual guides and beings of light. At the same time, the Merkaba serves as a powerful cleansing and vibrational harmonization mechanism, dissolving energetic blockages, balancing the chakras, and promoting a state of inner peace and well-being.

Finally, a fascinating aspect of this practice is the activation of spiritual DNA. Many spiritual traditions affirm that humans possess dormant layers of their genetic code that can be awakened through advanced energetic practices. The Merkaba, by connecting the individual to high frequencies, enhances this activation, facilitating the development of intuitive abilities, consciousness expansion, and alignment with one's life purpose.

By incorporating the Merkaba practice into a spiritual routine, one can experience a profound transformation, raising personal vibration and strengthening the connection with the universe.

40: Metatron's Cube

Metatron's Cube contains within it the five Platonic solids, which represent the elements of nature and the building blocks of reality. The Arcturians use Metatron's Cube to harmonize the subtle bodies, balance energies, and promote physical and emotional healing.

Metatron's Cube holds the five Platonic solids, symbolizing the fundamental elements of nature: earth, water, fire, air, and ether. Its sacred geometry acts as a catalyst for balance and healing, used by the Arcturians to harmonize the subtle bodies, stabilize energies, and support both physical and emotional healing.

To apply this powerful tool to yourself, it is essential to follow a structured process that allows for energetic attunement and the integration of its vibration into your personal field.

First, choose a quiet place where you can focus without interruptions. Sit comfortably, ensuring that your spine is straight and your feet are firmly planted on the ground. Close your eyes and begin deep, conscious breathing, gently inhaling through your nose and exhaling through your mouth, allowing your body to gradually relax. Visualize a golden light descending from above and surrounding you completely, filling you with serenity and protection.

With a calm mind and a receptive body, focus on activating Metatron's Cube. Imagine this sacred geometric structure forming in front of you, radiant in golden and blue hues. Feel its energy expanding, gently touching you and aligning with your vibration. Visualize the Cube slowly beginning to spin clockwise, emitting waves of pure energy that envelop your being. Allow yourself to feel this energy penetrating your field, dissolving tensions and balancing internal flows.

Now, direct your attention to the process of internal healing and balance. Visualize Metatron's Cube gently descending until it reaches your root chakra at the base of your spine. Let its energy strengthen your grounding and revitalize your life force. Then, move the structure to the sacral chakra, just below your navel, and perceive the activation of your creativity and emotional balance. At the solar plexus, the center of your confidence and personal power, imagine the Cube radiating an intense light, dissolving any blockages.

As it reaches the heart chakra, feel the Cube's energy expanding in waves of unconditional love and compassion. Let this light surround your chest, dissolving past wounds and opening the path for purer connections. Moving to the throat chakra, perceive the activation of your self-expression and inner truth, allowing your communication to become clearer and more authentic. At the third eye, located between your eyebrows, visualize the Cube enhancing your mental clarity and intuition, connecting you to deeper levels of perception. Finally, as it reaches the crown chakra at the top of your head, imagine a violet and golden light connecting you to the divine, bringing enlightenment and wisdom.

After this alignment, visualize the energy of the Cube expanding beyond your body, connecting with the universal field of wisdom. Feel your consciousness broadening, absorbing profound knowledge and insights. At this moment, mentally affirm: "I activate the sacred geometry of Metatron's Cube to purify, balance, and expand my energy."

To conclude, visualize the Cube slowing its rotation and gently settling within your energy field, where it will continue to vibrate in harmony with your essence. Take three deep breaths, feeling completely present and balanced. Slowly open your eyes, move gently, and return to your waking state with a renewed sense of well-being and clarity.

Beyond using it on yourself, Metatron's Cube can also be applied to others to promote healing and energetic balance. To do this, begin by creating a sacred space for the practice. Ask the person receiving the activation to sit or lie down comfortably, ensuring they are relaxed and in a receptive state. Guide them to breathe deeply, allowing their body and mind to open to the experience. Then, visualize a sphere of golden light surrounding both of you, forming an energetic field of protection and connection.

With the environment prepared, focus on activating Metatron's Cube over the person's body. Imagine it spinning gently above them, radiating healing energy and dissolving any blockages or accumulated density. If you intuitively feel the need, use your hands to direct this energy, channeling light over specific points and reinforcing the person's energy flow.

Now, visualize the Cube descending and positioning itself over each chakra, one at a time. At the root chakra, allow the Cube's energy to bring stability and strength. At the sacral chakra, envision a smooth flow of creativity and emotional balance being restored. At the solar plexus, feel the activation of personal power and self-confidence. As it reaches the heart chakra, allow the Cube to expand feelings of love and compassion. At the throat chakra, visualize an activation of genuine and authentic expression. At the third eye, sense the deepening of intuition, while at the crown chakra, envision a luminous spiritual expansion.

To enhance this process, specific crystals can be placed over each chakra, or vibrational frequencies such as 432 Hz or 528 Hz can be incorporated to support energetic harmonization.

When you feel the energy has stabilized, visualize Metatron's Cube anchoring itself within the person's auric field, where it will continue working on their balance. Ask them to take deep breaths and feel fully restored. To conclude, guide them through a brief meditation or recite a grounding mantra, such as: "May this sacred energy bring balance and clarity to my journey."

The benefits of this practice are profound and far-reaching. Beyond providing intense energetic harmonization, Metatron's Cube assists in aligning the chakras and subtle bodies, promoting a state of balance and overall well-being. Its vibration also supports access to higher states of consciousness, fostering greater connection with higher dimensions of knowledge and spirituality. Regular practice contributes to emotional healing, helping to release limiting patterns and restore mental clarity.

Ultimately, by activating this powerful sacred geometry, we not only protect and strengthen our energy field but also open ourselves to a journey of self-transformation and connection with the divine.

41: Spiral

The spiral is a symbol of growth, expansion, and evolution. It represents the movement of vital energy and the soul's journey toward ascension. The Arcturians use the spiral to activate DNA, accelerate the healing process, and promote a connection with universal wisdom.

The spiral is an ancient symbol of growth, expansion, and spiritual evolution, reflecting the flow of vital energy and the ascension of consciousness. Its movement resonates with the patterns of nature, from the rotation of galaxies to the growth of plants and the structure of human DNA itself. The Arcturians, beings known for their high consciousness and cosmic wisdom, use the spiral as a powerful tool for energetic activation, promoting the expansion of the self on different levels. By incorporating this symbol into spiritual practices, it is possible to accelerate healing processes, awaken dormant potentials, and establish a deep connection with universal wisdom.

To apply the spiral to yourself, the first step involves preparation and connection with this energy. Choose a quiet place where you can concentrate without interruptions. Sit comfortably or stand with your feet firmly aligned with the ground. Take a few deep breaths, allowing your mind and body to relax completely. Then, visualize a luminous spiral hovering above your head, radiating a vibrant and welcoming light that begins to gently descend toward you, preparing your energy field for activation.

As you move into the activation of the energy flow, imagine this spiral starting to rotate clockwise around your body. Feel its presence as a current of golden and bluish light completely enveloping you. Visualize this energy penetrating every cell, awakening cosmic memories, and activating your inner potential. Allow yourself to be carried by the sensation of lightness and expansion, noticing how your vibration rises and your energy field strengthens.

In the next stage, the activation of spiritual DNA, direct your attention to the center of your being, focusing on the heart chakra. Imagine a small golden spiral emerging at this point and beginning to expand, traveling throughout your body with its elevated frequency. Feel how this activation brings a wave of vitality, balance, and mental clarity. Allow this energy to dissolve blockages and open doors to the perception of new realities. To enhance this process, mentally affirm:

"The energy of the spiral activates my divine potential and awakens my inner wisdom."

Repeat it a few times, absorbing its meaning and allowing it to resonate deeply in your consciousness.

As you proceed to connect with universal wisdom, visualize the spiral expanding beyond the limits of your body, linking to the quantum field of the universe. Feel connected to an infinite source of knowledge and intuition. Allow this energy to bring subtle messages, insights, and energetic healing. Stay in this state for as long as you feel necessary, absorbing the vibration and allowing your consciousness to expand into new dimensions.

To conclude and integrate the experience, imagine the spiral slowing its rotation and stabilizing within your energy field. Take a deep breath and, as you exhale, bring your attention back to the present. Slowly open your eyes, noticing the feeling of balance and renewal. Move your body gently, allowing this new frequency to integrate fully into your being.

When applied to others, the spiral can act as a powerful channel for healing and vibrational elevation. The first step is to create a harmonious energetic space. Ask the person to sit or lie down comfortably and guide them to take deep breaths, fully relaxing. Visualize a field of light surrounding them, creating a safe and conducive environment for the experience.

Next, focus on visualization and energy direction. Imagine a large spiral of golden and bluish light appearing above the person and gently descending to envelop them. Visualize this spiral rotating clockwise around them, promoting energetic realignment. Direct this energy to balance the chakras, dissolve blockages, and restore harmony in the physical and spiritual field.

At the moment of DNA activation and consciousness expansion, visualize the spiral penetrating deeply into the person's cellular field. Mentally affirm that this activation awakens ancestral memories, intuitive abilities, and latent potentials. If you sense a specific area in need of healing or energetic adjustment, focus the spiral in that region, slowing its movement until harmonization is complete.

To integrate and anchor the effects of this practice, gradually slow down the spiral's rotation and visualize it stabilizing within the person's energy field. Guide them to take a few deep breaths, absorbing the new frequency and feeling fully connected. Conclude the process by chanting an alignment mantra or emitting high-vibration sounds, such as 741 Hz frequencies for cellular healing or 963 Hz for deepening spiritual connection.

The benefits of this practice are vast and encompass different levels of being. The activation of spiritual DNA promotes a profound inner awakening, while the harmonization of the energy field brings balance and well-being. By dissolving stagnant emotional and energetic patterns, the spiral aids in releasing blockages and expanding perception. This connection with cosmic forces accelerates healing processes and spiritual evolution, providing a journey of self-knowledge and transformation.

42: Mandala

Mandalas are geometric representations that symbolize wholeness and unity. They are used in meditation and healing practices to harmonize energy, calm the mind, and enhance concentration.

Mandalas are geometric representations that symbolize wholeness, balance, and unity. More than just shapes, they function as energetic portals that promote healing, concentration, and the expansion of consciousness. Their geometric structure, composed of symmetrical patterns, resonates with universal harmony, directly influencing the energy fields of those who use them. Ancient civilizations already understood this power and incorporated mandalas into rituals, temples, and spiritual practices. Among the Arcturians, beings highly evolved in both spirituality and technology, mandalas are essential tools for advanced meditations and energetic alignment. They understand that these sacred forms harmonize the subtle bodies, help calm the mind, and strengthen spiritual connection, allowing for a deeper attunement with higher frequencies.

The practical application of mandalas can be carried out in various ways, one of the most effective being meditation and the absorption of their energies. By using a mandala, whether physically or through mental visualization, it is possible to establish a vibrational field that directly affects the practitioner's energy. This process occurs through a continuous flow of resonance, where the mind and spirit align with the sacred geometry of the mandala, facilitating inner balance and expanded awareness.

To apply the mandala to yourself, the first step is preparation and selecting the right mandala. This initial moment is essential, as each mandala carries a specific vibration and should align with your current energy or the transformation you seek. The choice can be intuitive or based on a specific goal, such as healing, protection, energetic activation, or concentration. If using a printed or drawn mandala, place it in a visible location. If you prefer to visualize it, try to imagine its details and colors as clearly as possible. Then, settle into a quiet and comfortable place, adopt a relaxed posture, and begin a cycle of deep breathing, allowing your mind and body to enter a state of calm and receptivity.

In the second stage, the connection with the mandala begins. Gently fix your gaze on its center, letting your vision expand around the geometric patterns. If you are using a visualized mandala, imagine it slowly spinning in front of you, radiating energy in all directions. At this moment, attunement with the mandala begins to establish itself. Feel its vibration interacting with your energy field, allowing your consciousness to immerse itself in the details and colors of the image. This interaction creates an energy flow that helps harmonize emotions and thoughts, promoting a sense of alignment and inner balance.

The next stage involves the absorption and energetic alignment. Imagine the mandala starting to emit a soft, pulsating, and enveloping light that expands and integrates with your energy field. This light flows through your entire being, dissolving emotional blockages and unblocking energy channels. Visualize this energy purifying your chakras, restoring vitality, and strengthening your aura. Remain in this state for a few minutes, feeling increasingly lighter and vibrationally elevated. With each breath, allow this energy to intensify, revitalizing your mind and body.

Following this, the phase of integration and meditation begins. Gently close your eyes, maintaining the sensation of the mandala within you. Let this energy continue to manifest in all areas of your life. To enhance this process, mentally affirm:

"I integrate the harmony and balance of the mandala into all areas of my life."

Repeat this phrase mentally a few times, absorbing its intention. Feel how the mandala's energy adjusts within you, promoting a state of serenity and clarity. Remain in this meditative state for as long as you feel necessary, allowing your awareness to expand without haste.

Finally, it is time to return to a waking state and ground the absorbed energy. Slowly bring your attention back to your physical body. Gently move your hands, feet, and neck, feeling your connection with the surrounding environment. Open your eyes calmly and notice the sense of renewal and balance that the practice has provided. Feel gratitude for the experience and carry this positive energy throughout your day.

Beyond personal application, mandalas can also be used to benefit others. In this case, the first step is preparing the space and energy. Choose a mandala suited to the person's needs, whether for healing, protection, activation, or concentration. The environment should be quiet and free from external interference, allowing the recipient to deeply relax. Guide them to sit or lie down comfortably and begin deep breathing to induce a receptive state of relaxation.

The second step involves projecting the mandala into the person's energy field. Place the mandala near their body or visualize it gently spinning over their aura. Imagine this mandala emitting pulses of light that flow and fill their entire energy field, dissolving tension and restoring balance. If there is a specific area that requires harmonization, consciously direct the mandala's energy to that point, intensifying its effect.

After a few minutes of energetic interaction, it is time for stabilization and anchoring. Visualize the mandala harmoniously settling within the person's energy field, establishing a stable and revitalizing vibration. Guide them to visualize a soft light surrounding their entire being, bringing well-being and mental clarity. To conclude the practice, a mantra can be chanted, sealing the generated energy. An effective example is:

"Harmony and light flow through me, bringing peace and balance."

This affirmation strengthens the practice's effects and anchors the elevated vibration in the person receiving the mandala's energy.

The continuous use of mandalas brings numerous benefits to the body, mind, and spirit. Among their main positive effects are chakra and subtle body harmonization, enhanced concentration and mental focus, emotional balance, and stress reduction. Additionally, the practice aids in connecting with higher states of consciousness, allowing for a greater attunement with the higher self and the universe. Another fundamental aspect is the awakening of creativity and intuition, as mandalas act as catalysts for inner expression and expanded sensory perception.

By incorporating mandalas into your routine—whether through meditation, visualization, or energy harmonization—you open a powerful channel of connection with your higher essence. This simple yet profoundly transformative practice has the potential to elevate your vibration and bring a new level of balance to your life.

43: Meditation with Symbols

Meditating with Sacred Geometry symbols, such as the Flower of Life and the Merkaba, facilitates connection with the Arcturians, raises vibration, and promotes multidimensional healing.

Meditation with Sacred Geometry symbols is a deeply transformative practice capable of elevating vibration, facilitating connection with the Arcturians, and promoting multidimensional healing. These symbols act as energetic keys, unlocking portals of consciousness and harmonizing the subtle flows of being. Among the most powerful are the Flower of Life, which resonates with the fundamental structure of creation, and the Merkaba, a geometric light field that activates the Light Body and strengthens spiritual protection.

To apply this practice to yourself, it is essential to create an appropriate environment. Choose a quiet place where you can meditate without interruptions, ensuring a space of serenity and introspection. If desired, use sensory elements such as incense or essential oils to enhance the energetic harmony of the space. Sit comfortably, keeping your spine straight, your feet firmly on the ground, and your hands resting gently on your legs. Close your eyes and focus on your breathing, inhaling deeply through your nose and exhaling slowly through your mouth, allowing your body and mind to enter a state of deep relaxation.

Choosing the symbol is a crucial step, as each carries a specific frequency. If you select the Flower of Life, be aware that its energy promotes the activation of the energy field, universal connection, and cellular harmonization. The Merkaba, on the other hand, enhances spiritual ascension, strengthens energetic protection, and activates the Light Body. Visualize the symbol in front of you, shining with a golden luminosity, radiating subtle energy. Imagine this light gradually expanding until it envelops your entire being, filling every cell with its elevated vibration.

As the symbol glows before you, allow it to rotate gently, adjusting your vibrational frequency and realigning your chakras. Feel the energy flowing throughout your body, dissolving blockages and promoting healing on multiple levels. If you wish to deepen this connection, mentally repeat a powerful affirmation such as:

"Sacred Geometry activates my divine connection and elevates my consciousness."

This declaration reinforces the integration of the symbol's energy into your vibrational field, amplifying the effects of the practice.

Connection with the Arcturians can be activated by imagining the symbol's light projecting into a blue sphere of energy located above your head. This sphere represents a dimensional portal to higher frequencies. Visualize it gently expanding, establishing a communication channel with the Arcturians. Remain in this receptive state, opening yourself to messages, insights, and subtle sensations that may arise. Communication often occurs through deep intuitions or symbolic images, manifesting as a natural flow of cosmic understanding.

As you conclude the meditation, it is essential to anchor the experience to ensure energetic stability. Visualize the symbol's light gently fixing itself within your auric field, sealing the practice's benefits within you. Slowly bring your attention back to your physical body, feeling the contact with the ground, moving gently, and breathing deeply. Open your eyes and take a few moments to notice the subtle shifts in your energy before returning to your daily activities.

This same practice can be applied to others, promoting healing and energetic harmonization. To do this, start by preparing the recipient's energy field. Ask the person to lie down or sit comfortably and guide them to take deep breaths, allowing them to enter a state of relaxation. Mentally envision a blue sphere of light surrounding them, creating a safe and protected space for the meditation session.

The activation of the Sacred Geometry symbol should be done with clear intention. Choose the symbol best suited to the person's needs and visualize it positioned above them, radiating a gentle, healing light. Imagine it slowly rotating, emitting waves of energy that envelop the recipient's body, promoting balance and alignment.

To enhance the energy transmission, use your hands as channels for the symbol's energy. Feel the vibrational flow moving through you and intuitively sense which areas of the body need the most adjustment. If necessary, you may repeat a specific mantra or chant Arcturian activation sounds, intensifying the vibrational frequency of the healing process.

The integration of energy should be carried out gently. Visualize the symbol gradually diminishing in intensity, stabilizing within the person's energy field. Ask them to take a few deep breaths and, if desired, share their sensations and perceptions about the experience. Conclude the session with a statement of balance and harmony, such as:

"The light and harmony of Sacred Geometry flow freely in my life."

The benefits of this practice are vast and encompass multiple levels of being. Meditation with Sacred Geometry symbols enhances connection with higher dimensions, strengthens the energy field, and activates the Light Body. Additionally, it balances the chakras, promotes multidimensional healing, and expands intuition, facilitating access to cosmic information. As a result, it opens doors to a clearer and deeper communication with the Arcturians and other high-vibrational beings, fostering a spiritual alignment that resonates across all areas of life.

44: Visualization of Geometric Shapes

Visualizing geometric shapes, such as the spiral and Metatron's Cube, harmonizes the subtle bodies, promotes healing, and facilitates the manifestation of desires.

The practice of visualizing geometric shapes is a profound and transformative method capable of realigning the subtle bodies, promoting healing, and facilitating the manifestation of desires. Symbols like the spiral and Metatron's Cube carry vibrational frequencies that directly restructure the energy field, allowing for a deeper connection with higher states of consciousness. The Arcturians, beings known for their spiritual and technological advancement, use these shapes to adjust frequencies, balance energies, and create states of deep harmony, assisting those seeking to elevate their vibration and manifest intentions aligned with cosmic order.

To apply the visualization of geometric shapes to yourself, it is essential to follow a structured process. The first step is to create a suitable environment for the practice. Choose a quiet place where you can focus without interruptions. Sit comfortably or lie down, ensuring that your spine is aligned to allow proper energy flow. Take a few deep breaths, inhaling through your nose and exhaling slowly through your mouth, letting each exhalation release accumulated tension. Close your eyes and enter a receptive state, allowing your mind to become a fertile space for the energetic experience.

With your mind in a relaxed state, it is time to choose which geometric shape to visualize, depending on your goal. The spiral, for example, is ideal for expanding consciousness, cosmic connection, and DNA activation, while Metatron's Cube promotes energetic alignment, balance of the subtle bodies, and spiritual protection. Once you have chosen the shape, imagine it in front of you, composed of vibrant golden light, radiating energy that pulses gently in sync with the universe.

The next step is to integrate this geometric shape into your energy field. Visualize it slowly rotating as it approaches your body, gently passing through the layers of your auric field. Allow this energy to dissolve blockages and harmonize your frequencies, bringing balance and a deep sense of well-being. Feel this light penetrating every cell of your being, restructuring your energy and promoting healing where needed.

If you have a specific goal, such as achieving mental clarity, strengthening intuition, or manifesting a desire, direct the energy of the geometric shape toward that intention. See it expanding and emitting pulses of light that envelop your body, sending this vibration into the universe. Reinforce this connection with a powerful affirmation, such as:

"Sacred Geometry aligns my energy with the manifestation of my highest desires."

As you repeat this phrase mentally, feel the resonance of this energy co-creating your reality, adjusting to the universal field of abundance, and enabling the realization of your intentions.

To conclude the practice, visualize the geometric shape stabilizing in your aura, anchoring the energy so that its benefits endure. Breathe deeply, bringing your awareness back to the present moment. Move gently, feeling the integration of the experience before opening your eyes. This conclusion ensures that the process is absorbed in a balanced way, allowing you to continue with a sense of alignment and protection.

The visualization of geometric shapes can also be applied to others, aiding in the harmonization and healing of their energy fields. To do this, begin by preparing the environment and guiding the person to sit or lie down comfortably. Ask them to take deep breaths, allowing their body to relax gradually. Imagine a field of golden light surrounding them, creating a safe and harmonious space, ready to receive transformative energy.

Choose the appropriate symbol for the person's needs and visualize it positioned above them. See the geometric shape rotating gently, emitting waves of light that descend into their energy field. Direct this energy with intention, allowing it to dissolve blockages and realign frequencies. Intuitively observe which areas of the body need the most attention and mentally position the geometric shape over those regions.

If using Metatron's Cube, visualize it enveloping the person's entire body, balancing their chakras and deeply harmonizing their energy. If opting for the spiral, imagine it activating their spiritual DNA and awakening dormant potential. Allow yourself to feel the energy flowing, adjusting, and restoring energetic balance.

To complete the session, visualize the energy of the geometric shape gently stabilizing in the person's field, ensuring stability and continuity of the process. Ask them to take a few deep breaths and notice the feeling of balance and renewal. Reinforce the alignment with an affirmation such as:

"I integrate Sacred Geometry and allow my energy to flow in harmony with the cosmos."

This closure seals the practice and ensures that the energy remains active in the person's field, supporting their journey of healing and expansion.

The practice of visualizing geometric shapes offers numerous benefits, such as harmonizing the subtle bodies and balancing energy, facilitating physical and emotional healing. Additionally, this technique activates the energy of manifestation and co-creation, allowing intentions to materialize more fluidly. Another significant benefit is the expansion of perception, fostering a deeper connection with the Higher Self and facilitating access to elevated states of consciousness. Furthermore, spiritual protection and aura strengthening are reinforced, creating a more resilient and stable energy field against external adversities.

By incorporating this practice into your routine, you will continuously adjust your frequencies and align yourself with a more harmonious and elevated energetic flow. Sacred Geometry is a powerful tool that, when used with intention and regularity, can profoundly transform how we interact with our own energy and the universe.

45: Mandala Construction

Creating mandalas with specific colors and geometric shapes promotes emotional healing, creative expression, and connection with the Higher Self.

The construction of mandalas is a powerful practice for harmonizing emotions, expanding creativity, and strengthening the connection with subtle dimensions of consciousness. More than mere drawings or ornamental shapes, mandalas act as energetic portals, channeling specific frequencies through colors and sacred geometries. Various ancient cultures and spiritual traditions have long recognized their influence on inner balance and the activation of elevated states of perception. The Arcturians, beings known for their wisdom and advanced technology, use this technique to adjust vibrations, stabilize the energy field, and stimulate consciousness expansion. By creating a mandala, you not only express your artistic intuition but also establish a sacred energy field, aligning yourself with the cosmic flow and allowing your intention to materialize through shapes and colors that resonate with your essence.

The process of creating a personal mandala begins with a moment of introspection and preparation. Choose a quiet environment where you can focus without interruptions. The atmosphere should promote relaxation, and you may include incense, candles, or soft music if desired. Take a few deep breaths, allowing your mind to calm and your body to enter a receptive state. This is the time to set your mandala's intention, which may relate to

Emotional healing – working through traumas, anxiety, and seeking inner balance.

Consciousness expansion – fostering a deeper connection with the Higher Self and awakening intuitive faculties.

Manifestation of desires – attracting opportunities and transforming limiting patterns.

With your intention defined, the choice of colors and geometric shapes becomes an essential step, as each carries a specific vibration.

Blue evokes peace, mental clarity, and spiritual protection.

Green is linked to healing, regeneration, and emotional balance.

Gold symbolizes spiritual elevation, enlightenment, and connection with higher planes.

Purple supports consciousness expansion, intuition, and energetic transmutation.

In addition to colors, geometric shapes play a fundamental role in the mandala's energetic structure:

The Flower of Life promotes energetic alignment and universal harmony.

The Spiral represents evolution, the continuous flow of energy, and DNA activation.

Metatron's Cube offers protection, balance, and energetic purification.

Mandalas can be created using various mediums, such as paper, canvas, colored sand, or even digital tools, depending on your preference and skill. The process begins with a central point, symbolizing the connection with the Universe and the Higher Self. From this point, geometric patterns and symmetrical shapes are drawn, radiating outward in a continuous flow. There is no need to follow a rigid plan—allow your intuition to guide your choice of colors and forms, letting energy naturally flow through the art.

Once completed, the mandala needs to be energetically activated to amplify its vibration. To do this, place your hands over it and close your eyes, visualizing a stream of golden light descending from the cosmos and infusing your creation with elevated energy. While maintaining this connection, mentally affirm:

"This mandala carries the energy of healing and balance, aligning me with universal harmony."

Allow this vibration to integrate into your energy field, feeling the subtle presence of the mandala working within you.

Using the mandala continuously strengthens its influence in your life. Place it in a visible location, such as an altar, a wall, or a sacred space, so its energy remains active. Whenever you need balance or guidance, focus on the mandala, allowing its frequency to interact with your energy field. If you feel the mandala has fulfilled its purpose, you may dissolve it symbolically—burning it (if on paper) or dismantling it—releasing its energy back into the universe.

Creating mandalas for others is an act of energetic giving and elevated intention. Before starting, it is important to define the intention and attune yourself to the energy of the recipient. To do this, ask them about their desired goal—whether healing, protection, expansion, or manifestation—and, if possible, have them share emotions or life areas needing balance. Take deep breaths and visualize an energetic link between you and them, allowing intuition to guide the creative process.

While drawing or painting, personalize the mandala according to their needs, selecting colors and shapes that resonate with their vibrational field. As you work, visualize frequencies of light flowing into the mandala, infusing it with healing and harmonizing energy. To finalize, add a central point of golden light, representing balance, protection, and completeness.

The activation of a mandala for another person follows a similar ritual to a personal mandala. Place your hands over it and visualize a blue and golden sphere of energy surrounding it, channeling your intention into the creation. Mentally affirm:

"This mandala channels healing and balancing energy for [name of the person], assisting them on their path."

Then, send the mandala to the person and guide them on how to use it—whether by displaying it in a special place, meditating with it, or focusing on it regularly.

Benefits of Mandala Construction

The practice of creating mandalas brings profound and far-reaching benefits:

Energetic harmonization – helps release repressed emotions, allowing emotional and mental purification.

Enhanced creativity and intuition – fosters the expression of inner essence and intuitive flow.

Spiritual healing and connection – strengthens the bond with the Higher Self and promotes self-awareness.

Manifestation and intention alignment – supports the attraction of aligned opportunities and transformation of limiting patterns.

By incorporating mandala construction into your routine, you create a sacred space for personal exploration, self-healing, and deep connection with the universe. This practice is a powerful tool for transformation, allowing you to realign your energy, elevate your vibration, and integrate the wisdom of Sacred Geometry into your life.

46: Use of Crystals

Combining crystals with sacred geometric shapes amplifies healing energy and directs it toward a specific purpose.

The combination of crystals with sacred geometric shapes is an ancient practice that enhances healing energy and channels it toward a specific goal. The Arcturians use this technique to adjust vibrational patterns, activate energy healing processes, and expand consciousness. Each crystal carries a unique frequency, which can be intensified when aligned with geometric structures such as Metatron's Cube, the Flower of Life, and the Merkaba.

To apply this technique to yourself, it is essential to follow a structured process. First, you must define the intention to be worked on and choose the corresponding crystal. Clear quartz is ideal for purification and energetic balance; amethyst promotes spiritual protection and intuition; black tourmaline provides cleansing of dense energies and grounding; rose quartz aids in emotional healing and harmony; and selenite raises vibration and connects with higher dimensions. At the same time, the choice of sacred geometry will amplify the crystal's energy: Metatron's Cube acts in protection and balance of the subtle bodies, the Flower of Life harmonizes and activates vital energy, and the Merkaba promotes Light Body activation and spiritual ascension.

After this selection, preparing the environment and the crystal becomes essential. The space should be calm, free of external interference. The crystal needs to be purified before use, which can be done by passing it through incense smoke, exposing it to sunlight or moonlight, or, if safe for that type of crystal, immersing it in saltwater. Holding the crystal, you must set the intention for the energy you wish to activate, focusing on the established purpose.

Energy activation occurs when the crystal is placed on a representation of sacred geometry, which can be a drawing, a mat, or a mental visualization. Sitting comfortably, close your eyes and take deep breaths. Imagine the crystal emitting an intense light that forms the geometry around your body. This energy expands, flowing through all the chakras and dissolving energetic blockages.

Directing the energy is a crucial step. For emotional healing, the crystal should be placed over the heart chakra, visualizing a pink light filling the heart. For protection and grounding, place the crystal at the base of the spine or in your hands, imagining a golden light enveloping your entire energy field. If the goal is consciousness expansion, the crystal should be held at the level of the third eye, visualizing a portal of light opening.

The process should be concluded carefully to ensure energetic integration. After feeling the energy being absorbed, take three deep breaths before slowly opening your eyes. Expressing gratitude to the crystal and the sacred geometry is an important gesture to seal the connection. The crystal should be stored in a special place and, if possible, left on the sacred geometry to maintain its high vibration.

This technique can also be applied to others, following a similar procedure. First, the space and the recipient should be prepared. The person can lie down or sit comfortably, taking deep breaths to relax. Creating a field of light around them ensures protection and harmony during the process.

When selecting crystals, it is necessary to consider the person's energetic needs and place them on the main chakras or strategic points of the body. A drawing of sacred geometry can be placed under the recipient or mentally visualized around them, creating a structure of energetic support.

Activation and energy flow happen when the crystals are imagined emitting waves of light that expand throughout the person's energy field. In the case of Metatron's Cube, the crystals can be visualized forming this structure around the body, promoting protection and balance. The Flower of Life, on the other hand, can be imagined pulsating and restoring the flow of vital energy.

To deepen healing and integration, it is recommended to gently pass the hands over the crystals, directing energy to the recipient's auric field. The person can be encouraged to feel the subtle changes in their body and emotions. The use of sound frequencies, such as 432 Hz or 852 Hz, can intensify energetic harmonization.

The process should be concluded by gently removing the crystals and guiding the recipient to take a few deep breaths. It is important for them to move slowly before standing up to ensure proper grounding. To finalize, a balancing affirmation can be used, such as: "I am in harmony with the flow of the universe, and my energy is aligned with the highest good."

The benefits of this practice are numerous. Using crystals with sacred geometry amplifies healing energy, balances the chakras and subtle bodies, provides spiritual protection, facilitates the manifestation of intentions and desires, and deepens the connection with the Higher Self and the Arcturians.

47: Healing with Hands

Using the hands to trace Sacred Geometry symbols over the patient's body promotes energetic harmonization and physical and emotional healing. Healing with hands, used to trace Sacred Geometry symbols over the patient's body, is a powerful energetic harmonization technique that works on both the physical and emotional levels. The Arcturians, beings known for their advanced spiritual wisdom, apply this method to restore the flow of the vibrational field, dissolve energetic blockages, and reconnect individuals with their cosmic essence. When symbols such as the Merkaba, the Flower of Life, and Metatron's Cube are projected onto the body, a profound energetic reconfiguration occurs, facilitating healing and the activation of spiritual DNA, allowing individuals to access higher states of consciousness and balance.

To apply this technique to yourself, it is essential to follow a careful process, ensuring that the energy flows freely and fulfills its restorative function. The first step involves energetic preparation: find a quiet, undisturbed place and adopt a comfortable position, keeping your spine straight and feet aligned with the ground. Closing your eyes, begin a cycle of deep breathing, allowing the mind to calm and the body to become receptive to subtle energy. Next, visualize a golden light descending from the universe and surrounding your entire body, creating a field of protection and energetic activation.

Choosing the appropriate symbol is the next step and should be done according to your current needs. The Merkaba, for instance, is ideal for Light Body activation and energetic protection, while the Flower of Life aids in cellular harmonization and emotional balance. Metatron's Cube is especially useful for purification and alignment of the subtle bodies, while the Spiral promotes DNA activation and maintains a continuous energy flow. With the chosen symbol in mind, begin the energetic tracing. Moving your hands gently over your auric field, visualize the symbol being drawn in the air with golden and blue light emanating from your hands. This visualization is not merely symbolic but directly affects the energetic field, dissolving blockages and restoring vibrational harmony.

After tracing the symbol, the energy is intensified by placing your hands over the area that requires healing, such as the heart, solar plexus, or head. Visualizing the symbol expanding and filling your entire being with light strengthens its restorative effect. To enhance the impact, an affirmation can be mentally repeated, such as: "Sacred Geometry restores my balance and activates my connection with the divine source." This moment is crucial for consolidating energetic changes and integrating the benefits of the practice.

The process should be concluded gradually, reducing the intensity of the visualization and allowing the energy to stabilize. Deep breathing and gentle body movements help reintegrate into the physical state. It is essential to express gratitude for the established connection and energetic restoration before fully ending the practice.

When applied to others, healing with hands requires special attention to the preparation of the environment and the patient. The space should be harmonious, quiet, and free from external interference. The patient can be guided to lie down or sit comfortably and take deep breaths, entering a receptive state of relaxation. Creating a sphere of golden and blue light around both the healer and the patient helps establish a safe energetic field for the healing session.

The choice of the Sacred Geometry symbol should consider the person's specific needs, just as in self-healing. Positioning your hands over the patient's body without directly touching them, visualize the symbol emerging in their auric field. The symbol can then be drawn in the air above the area that needs healing, allowing its vibration to integrate into the patient's energy field.

Energy direction occurs as waves of light emanate from your hands and are absorbed by the person's body. During this process, you may notice areas of resistance or energetic blockages. If necessary, the symbol can be redrawn or repositioned to intensify harmonization and ensure a more effective vibrational adjustment. Intuition plays a fundamental role at this stage, guiding the healer to make necessary adjustments based on the patient's energetic response.

Once the healing feels complete, integration and stabilization of the energy are essential. The projected symbol should be gently anchored in the person's energy field, ensuring its effect endures. To assist in assimilation, the patient can be encouraged to take deep breaths and internalize the received energy. An integration affirmation, such as "This healing energy restores my harmony and activates my alignment with the Universe," can be used to reinforce the effects of the session.

The closing should be done carefully to ensure the energy stabilizes harmoniously. Passing your hands gently around the patient's body helps consolidate the healing and prevent energetic dispersion. Before standing up, the patient should be encouraged to move slowly, promoting proper grounding. As a final step, the healer should wash their hands or rinse them under running water to release any energetic residue absorbed during the practice.

The benefits of healing with hands and Sacred Geometry are vast and profoundly impact physical, emotional, and spiritual health. This method restores energetic balance, releasing blockages and misaligned vibrational patterns. Additionally, it promotes the activation of spiritual DNA and the Light Body, strengthening the connection with higher dimensions and facilitating consciousness awakening. Harmonization of the chakras and subtle bodies creates a state of overall well-being, allowing vital energy to flow more evenly and healthily.

The consistent practice of this technique not only promotes self-healing but also expands energetic sensitivity and the ability to assist others in their harmonization process. Through the conscious use of sacred symbols and focused intention, it is possible to transform the vibrational field, restoring harmony and activating the healing potential present in every being.

48: Frequencies of Light and Sound

Using frequencies of light and sound that resonate with Sacred Geometry patterns amplifies healing power and promotes the harmonization of the subtle bodies. The use of light and sound frequencies aligned with Sacred Geometry enhances healing power and facilitates the harmonization of the subtle bodies. Each frequency resonates with a specific energetic aspect, activating higher states of consciousness and promoting physical, emotional, and spiritual healing. The Arcturians, beings known for their high level of spiritual and technological development, employ this technique to recalibrate the vibrational field, dissolve energetic blockages, and expand individuals' cosmic perception. Specific sounds and light patterns associated with Sacred Geometry aid in the reactivation of spiritual DNA and strengthen the connection with higher dimensions, allowing for a deep alignment with the energies of the universe.

To apply this technique to yourself, the first step is choosing the sound frequency and the Sacred Geometry symbol. Each frequency carries a specific purpose:
- 396 Hz helps release fears and emotional blockages,

- 432 Hz promotes universal harmony and energetic balance,
- 528 Hz is known for its ability to regenerate cells and activate DNA,
- 741 Hz works in energetic cleansing and protection against negative vibrations,
- 963 Hz expands consciousness, facilitating the connection with the Higher Self.

Alongside the choice of frequency, selecting a geometric symbol enhances vibrational effects. The Flower of Life sustains the balance of the energy field and connection with the universal matrix, while Metatron's Cube offers energetic protection and alignment of the subtle bodies. The Merkaba assists in Light Body activation and spiritual ascension, while the Spiral favors the expansion of vital energy and the harmonic flow of consciousness.

After making the appropriate selection, the next step is preparation and attunement to the frequency. Finding a quiet and comfortable place is essential to creating an ideal environment for the practice. If possible, listening to the chosen frequency through headphones or speakers ensures full immersion. With the body relaxed, sit or lie down, close your eyes, and take several deep breaths. During this process, imagination plays a fundamental role: visualizing a wave of vibrant light descending from the universe and enveloping the body with its subtle and healing energy enhances the experience.

The integration of Sacred Geometry and sound vibration occurs when the geometric symbol is visualized gently rotating above the head, radiating its energy. The resonance with the sound frequency should be felt in every cell of the body, allowing waves of light and sound to expand and align the chakras, dissolving any energetic blockages. Remaining in this state of energetic reception, feeling the vibrational flow and absorbing the subtle frequencies, is essential for the benefits to be fully integrated.

The next stage involves expanding consciousness and deepening the spiritual connection. At this moment, the sound frequency transforms into geometric patterns filling the surrounding space, creating an energetic web that amplifies perception. Consciousness gradually expands, connecting with the universal field of cosmic wisdom. To anchor this connection, the following affirmation can be mentally repeated: "Sacred Geometry and sound vibration harmonize my being and expand my consciousness."

At the end of the practice, a moment of stabilization and energetic grounding is necessary. Visualizing the energy consolidating within the auric field helps integrate vibrational effects. Deep breathing and bringing awareness to the present moment are crucial to avoiding any feeling of disorientation. Before opening the eyes, it is recommended to move the body gently to ensure proper grounding, allowing the experience to serve as a solid foundation for energetic balance.

When this technique is applied to others, preparing the environment and the recipient is essential. The person should be guided to lie down or sit comfortably while the chosen sound frequency is played at a soft volume, creating an immersive and harmonizing sound field. Visualizing a sphere of vibrant light around the patient establishes a protected healing field where energy can flow in a balanced way.

The activation of Sacred Geometry occurs through the selection of an appropriate geometric symbol for the process. It should be visualized above the person, radiating pulsating light in sync with the used sound frequency. This luminous and vibrational emission directs its energy to different areas of the body, promoting balance and subtle realignment.

To amplify energy and enhance vibrational healing, the practitioner may use their hands to sense areas of blockages or regions needing a greater energetic flow. Intention and mental focus play a crucial role: visualizing the sound frequency dissolving negative patterns or misaligned vibrations strengthens the technique's potency. If desired, vocalizing tones, such as the sounds "OM" or "AH," can intensify the resonance of healing, amplifying the connection with higher energies.

The integration and conclusion of the session occur when the sound and geometric energy stabilize within the patient's auric field. To consolidate the therapeutic effects, the person can be encouraged to take deep breaths and feel the harmony within themselves. Ending with an integration affirmation, such as "Sound and light restore my balance and align me with the flow of the universe," reinforces the connection with the healing vibration.

Finally, grounding and returning to normal consciousness are crucial to ensuring the person fully returns to a wakeful state. It is recommended to guide them to move gently before standing up to prevent dizziness or energetic dispersion. Drinking a glass of water can aid in grounding and stabilizing the energy field. Additionally, the practitioner can wash their hands or use grounding crystals, such as hematite or black onyx, to rebalance their own energy after the session.

The benefits of using light and sound frequencies are vast and deeply transformative. This practice elevates vibrational frequency and harmonizes the energy field, promoting overall well-being. Additionally, it facilitates the release of emotional and energetic blockages, allowing energy to flow more freely and harmoniously. The expansion of perception and activation of spiritual DNA strengthen the connection with higher dimensions and the Arcturians, enabling a deeper alignment with cosmic consciousness. Finally, this practice contributes to energetic protection and environmental purification, creating spaces of harmony and vibrational balance.

By integrating these techniques into daily life, it becomes possible to experience a new level of consciousness and well-being, anchoring in physical reality the elevated vibrations that resonate with universal harmony.

49: Geometry in Our Life

Integrating Sacred Geometry into our daily lives is more than a symbolic act; it is a way to align our energy with the patterns that govern all of creation. When we choose to incorporate these principles into our routines—whether through the arrangement of furniture in our homes, the selection of clothing and accessories with geometric symbols, or even in spiritual and meditative practices—we are, in fact, connecting with a universal language that transcends time and space. This subtle alignment influences not only our individual energy field but also the harmony of the environments we inhabit and the people around us.

The connection with Sacred Geometry allows us to perceive that everything in the universe vibrates at specific frequencies, and each geometric shape carries a unique vibrational signature. The Arcturians teach that when these patterns are consciously integrated into our daily lives, they help realign our energy, restoring the natural balance of body and mind. Thus, when we meditate in front of a symbol like the Flower of Life or use Metatron's Cube in practices of protection and spiritual elevation, we are activating frequencies that harmonize our energy with cosmic rhythms.

Beyond meditative practices, the presence of Sacred Geometry in our environment can completely transform our perception and well-being. Architectures inspired by these principles use harmonic proportions and specific geometric forms to create spaces that foster balance and high vibrational energy. The arrangement of furniture and objects in a space can be adjusted to reflect geometric patterns such as the Fibonacci Sequence or the Golden Ratio, creating a sense of flow and well-being. Mandalas, fractals, and geometric patterns can be incorporated into walls, floors, or even small decorative details to intensify the energy of the place.

This influence of Sacred Geometry also extends to how we express ourselves in the world. Wearing sacred symbols, carrying geometric jewelry and amulets, or even using vibrational patterns in personal accessories is a way to maintain a constant resonance with these elevated frequencies. Many believe that these symbols not only provide protection but also expand consciousness and facilitate deeper spiritual connections.

By incorporating Sacred Geometry into our lives, we open ourselves to a continuous flow of balance and expansion. This journey of reconnection leads us to a heightened sensitivity and awareness of the subtle forces around us, allowing us to understand our interconnection with all of creation. Thus, harmony and healing cease to be abstract concepts and become lived experiences, reflected in every conscious choice we make. In this way, we co-create a reality where the sacred is not separate from the everyday but rather woven into every moment of our existence, transforming the way we see and interact with the world around us.

Epilogue

And now?

You have traveled through these pages as one who walks a path of revelations. You have left behind doubts, absorbed teachings, and, more than anything, experienced a new way of perceiving yourself and the universe. But know this: this is not an endpoint. It is, in truth, a gateway to infinite possibilities.

The knowledge that has reached you cannot be stored as a mere memory or treated as a distant concept. It pulses within every cell of your energetic body. It vibrates in the subtlety of your thoughts. It manifests in every decision you make from this moment forward.

You have understood that healing is not an isolated event but a continuous flow. That your energy responds to every intention, every word, every choice. And, above all, that you hold in your hands the power to transform your reality—not through effort, but through the vibrational awareness you now carry.

The Arcturians, these benevolent guides, will continue to send you signs. An unexpected synchronicity. A profound insight in the midst of silence. A growing sense of belonging each day. You are no longer the same as when you began this reading.

Your frequency has shifted. Your perception has expanded.

But what will you do with this?

Apply it. Integrate it. Practice it.

With every breath, remember that your energy is your most powerful language. Cultivate the harmony taught here, experiment with the techniques, explore your spiritual connection. Allow yourself to continue expanding, for the journey of awakening has no end—only new beginnings.

And when you feel the need for a reminder, a confirmation, or a push forward, return to these pages. They will be here, alive, waiting to resonate with your evolution.

You are not alone. You never were.

The universe watches.

Your being vibrates.

And the journey continues.

www.ingramcontent.com/pod-product-compliance
Lightning Source LLC
LaVergne TN
LVHW040045080526
838202LV00045B/3500